Constructing Patienthood in Brokered Medical Interaction

Constructing Patienthood in Brokered Medical Interaction

Iraqi–English Encounters

Afaf Ali

LEXINGTON BOOKS
Lanham • Boulder • New York • London

Published by Lexington Books
An imprint of The Rowman & Littlefield Publishing Group, Inc.
4501 Forbes Boulevard, Suite 200, Lanham, Maryland 20706
www.rowman.com

86-90 Paul Street, London EC2A 4NE

British Library Cataloguing in Publication Information Available

Library of Congress Cataloging-in-Publication Data Available

ISBN: 978-1-66690-238-9 (cloth)
ISBN: 978-1-66690-239-6 (electronic)

Contents

List of Figures and Tables

FIGURES

TABLES

Acknowledgments

Over the years, I mediated the American language and culture to many immediate members of my family after they arrived in California, leaving our home country, Iraq. I translated their oral and written communications in various contexts, such as immigration, healthcare, employment, apartment renting, and education. Not all activities required language translation only. On many occasions, I had to broker American social norms and institutional cultures.

A specific experience at a doctor's office had a profound impact on my research directions. I recall feeling a sense of discomfort when the doctor asked me to "tell your father he is very smart for bringing these old medical records." I felt his act, or perhaps his tone, of casting an unsolicited evaluation for the simple deed of bringing medical records to a first-time establishing-care visit was a bit presumptuous. I was positioned to transfer to my father this verdict about his cognitive capacity.

What I performed at that clinic and elsewhere is identified as *language brokering*; and I was the *language broker*. Learning the dominant language and culture is one of the first obstacles immigrants face in their resettlement journey. The difficulty stems from the fact that integration is not a linear acculturation process but a set of complex experiences that vary according to when and where daily interactions occur. For example, conversing in healthcare clinics requires a set of cultural norms and vocabulary items that differ from those used in a teacher–parent conference, shopping malls, or casual conversations at home.

I have examined the Arab American experience among a sample of college-age language brokers by employing interviewing and survey methods. Here, I study brokered medical interactions between Iraqi patients and U.S. healthcare providers using the method of conversation analysis. I examine the verbal and nonverbal actions of patients—like my father, who depends on family members—like me, to translate their medical interactions. The work is situated within the U.S.'s Arab American community, to which I belong, but the study design and findings may be applicable to mediated dominant-limited languages medical encounters in general.

The project has benefited from the intellect of prominent scholars in the field of language brokering, social interaction, and Arabic studies during my graduate years and after. I learned about language brokering from a first-year graduate seminar with Marjorie F. Orellana. As I witnessed her passion and insightful views, I knew this subject will be the thing to occupy my mind. Similarly, from the first social-interaction course meeting with John Heritage and Steven Clayman at the UCLA Department of Sociology, I was hooked on thinking and seeing the achievements of micro-actions. To the Goodwins, Candy, and Chuck, I owe a world of gratitude for everything I know and ponder upon regarding human actions has started in a lecture with one of them. Michael Cooperson inspired what I know about Arabic teaching, guided me through Arabic transliteration, and then *this* "put in your sentence only what needs to be there." As a project co-chair jointly with Charles Goodwin, Katrina Daly Thompson shaped my thinking about multilingualism and language communication. To her, I am dutifully grateful.

The work is dedicated to participating families, kindly acknowledging and appreciating the generosity by which they opened their homes and lives to usher in my journey into medical interactional research. This work is also dedicated to all immigrant families, humbled by the realities they endure in pursuing a better life for their families, to their children and mine, Sami, Naida and Dalia.

Introduction

Language Brokering—Terms and Conditions

Language brokering is translating oral and written texts by nonprofessional persons, a practice that has submerged into a wide interdisciplinary research ground since the mid-1990s motivated by the vast mobility of world populations. The practice is mostly associated with the intermediatory work of bilingual children on the behalf of their monolingual family members. This chapter informs the reader about the primary scholarly conversations as an entry into this complicated social, linguistic, and cognitive practice. Then, it elaborates on critical issues related to cross-linguistic doctor–patient interactions mediated by professional and nonprofessional interpreters.

The number of people with limited language proficiency who speak languages other than English at home is steadily growing. According to the 2019 U.S. Census Bureau report, about 68 million, almost one in five, speak a foreign language at home, a leap from one in ten in 1980, with 16.3 percent of this population speaking English "not well" and 5.3 percent "do not speak English at all." Concerning the Arabic American community, 3.7 million Arabic speakers live in the United States as reported by the Arab American Institute (n.d.). The community consists of considerably younger population with only 13 percent 60 years or older, also characterized by a high number of professionals and business owners, mostly naturalized citizens; yet still, 35 percent of the population leverage "less than very well" English skills, though these numbers could vary by sources. When seeking medical care, these individuals interact with a system built for and run by English speakers. Their communications may be facilitated formally by certified medical interpreters or informally by ad hoc bilinguals and family members. Among these two modes of communication—professional and nonprofessional interpretation—professional interpretation has relished a longer research trajectory within the fields of translation, linguistics, and bilingual studies. The linguistic and cultural practice of nonprofessional interpretation among immigrant families also has captured growing scholarly interest under many terms, one of which is the term adopted in this book, language brokering (LB).

The work of language brokers, even those with high levels of bilingual proficiency, differs from the work of professional interpreters considerably. Language brokers are taken care by, or they care for, those who use their interpretation. They are personally invested in the practice's details and outcomes. When translating, they often align themselves with family members, while professional interpreters conduct their translation in accordance with institutional regulations. The type of knowledge and sense of responsibility of each group influence the ways in which information is transferred between limited-English speakers and members of the dominant society. Whereas professional translators receive training in a specific domain, such as court or medical interpretation, language brokers perform these services in varied settings without any formal training other than their own accumulated experiences. Even within the same domain, demands of translation differ a great deal. For example, brokering a routine medical visit to a primary-care doctor differs from brokering interactions in a specialist clinic or emergency rooms. Studies have reported that language brokering happens almost in all aspects of everyday life, such as at home, schools, police stations, post offices, shopping malls, hospitals and clinics, pharmacies, and even car rides to help with directions.

Another point of departure is age and related issues. Whereas professional interpreters are working adults, language brokers may be of any age. Studies suggest that most immigrant individuals experience language brokering at some point regardless of age or bilingual abilities and may continue to do so as adults (Tse, 1995, 1996; Valdés, 2003; Weisskirch, 2006). Finally, professionals are often specialized in a specific fields of translation, such as conference interpretation or literary translation, whereas children of immigrant families translate all types of communicational modes, including oral, written, media, and online materials. While mending language and cultural disparities, language brokers gain intercultural and translanguaging skills (García-Sánchez & Orellana, 2022), which may advance the educational sector (Donner et al., 2007). They also form a bridge between domestic and institutional cultures and benefit the general labor and economic conditions when they facilitate interactions between their families and healthcare providers, officials, merchants, and others (Katz, 2014; Orellana et al., 2001). Their experiences start at home so that they reflect household functions, rather than institutional ideologies. Vikki Katz (2014) argues that language brokering is shaped by domestic features, making home environments central to how immigrant families deal with the dominant culture. On the account, language brokers tailor serves to the needs of the served.

For valid reasons, most language brokering research is primarily concerned with the language broker's well-being and development. Although this chief concern is justified, it brackets most of the produced knowledge on one side of the story, leaving the other side largely untold. Before further unpacking the LB research, I will discuss next an issue of terminology that, as I view it, has had a no-small impact on research directions.

A TERMINOLOGY ISSUE

A number of terms have been used to study the translation practices among and for members of immigrant communities, some of which are: natural translation (Harris, 1973), family interpreting (Valdés, 2003), paraphrasing (Orellana et al., 2003), community interpretation (Angelelli, 2004), the activity of children translation among immigrant families (Wadensjö, 1995), child brokering (Katz, 2014b), and cultural brokering (Jones & Trickett, 2005). Each one of these terms highlights a certain angle of the practice; albeit the term language brokering has been employed to cover a wider range of anthropological, psychological, and linguistic perspectives. It foregrounds a sense of navigating elements of intersubjectivity, translanguaging, and interculturality as shaped and reshaped by accumulated experiences (García-Sánchez, 2010; García-Sánchez & Orellana, 2022).

Early employment of the term appeared in a two-year ethnography by Sheila Shannon (1987), a researcher with background in education and anthropology, to examine bilingual practices among Latino children. Soon after, a couple of articles discussed the ways in which U.S. Chinese and Vietnamese families adjust to the demands of a new host country through the translation of their children (McQuillan & Tse, 1995; Tse, 1995, 1996). A catalyst juncture in the field development came with a two-year multisite ethnography by Marjorie F. Orellana, which became the basis for multiple publications individually and with associates and has contributed to drawing wide attention to the multifaceted work of bilingual children in minority communities (Orellana, 2001; Orellana et al. 2001, 2003, 2009, 2015; Orellana et al., 2003; García-Sánchez & Orellana, 2006; Guan et al., 2016). Currently, LB research covers diverse scholarships from the fields of communication, education, anthropology, sociology, linguistics, psychology, and neuroscience.

The practice is defined as "the work that the children of immigrants do as they use their skills in two languages to read, write, listen, speak, and do things for their families" (Orellana, 2009, p. 1), with the word children referring to persons from different age groups. LB can be found commonly practiced among intergenerational family members when bilinguals translate between older and younger monolingual relatives, but academic concerns are widely interested in examining associative psychological and cognitive impacts of language brokering on participants. A large part of the relevant fields also study elements that facilitate the process of meaning-making between two different world views and customs. The utility of the terms language broker or child broker reflects the primary perspective through which scholars have dealt with the practice, mainly through a focal interest in the mediator's side. The person who depends on the brokering act is addressed either in relation to the interactional setting (e.g., patient, asylum seeker, shopper) or in kinship terms (e.g., mother, father, grandparents). Insofar as the research coinage is concerned, the person managing personal matters in the LB contact zones is identified by settings or relations rather than their role or agency.

To situate the novice speaker within the practice regardless of settings or relationships, I have coined the term *language brokeree*. The expression is directed to conceptualize the actions of the limited-in-the-dominant-language speaker in ways similar to the applications of the term, the language broker. My objective for the term is threefold: first, to situate the language brokeree on an equal analytical footing with the language broker as interactional partners, and second to resolve an issue of referencing in which language proficiency is used as an addressee form. Since LB participants differ widely in their comprehension and speaking abilities, scholars are unconcerned with assessing language proficiencies; they primarily acknowledge the work of immigrant families who agentively incorporate LB in quotidian communications. Finally, designating a term when referring to individuals with various identities and brokering needs may act as a curser to coalesce, and therefore advance, knowledge produced by diverse fields and perspectives. Accordingly, I define the language brokeree as an individual with various levels of linguistic and cultural competencies who solicits the help of bilingual individuals, often family members, to mend communicational problems in casual and institutional settings of the dominant society.

LANGUAGE BROKERING RESEARCH

The early anecdotes of children's translation came from linguists documenting the speaking abilities of their bilingual children, which were analyzed and identified as *Natural Translation* by Brian Harris, a Canadian scholar of linguistics and translation and an English-Arabic interpreter. These precursor studies mentioned children's translation in passing as a part of bilingual development and not necessarily a separate phenomenon of its own right. Increasingly, children's translation began to be recognized for its social purposes, a developing strategy that facilitates vital affairs in novel environments. Through translation, children have contributed to their families' integration and assimilation since the first waves of immigration in ways far less acknowledged and recognized in the relevant literature.

The practice is often perceived differently depending on how the notion of childhood is defined. The Western culture views child brokering as a form of adult-like responsibility with age-inappropriate constraints. Immigrant families, however, frame the act broadly as a way of managing familial affairs, unnecessarily associated with losing parents' authority or empowering children inappropriately. These opposite standpoints on children's translation have been presented mostly in terms of advantages and disadvantages.

Review studies are a valid indicator of research development. Shen et al. (2017) reviewed twenty-seven articles to examine LB in the light of related social variables, which they organized into six dimensions: socioemotional (depression and internalized symptoms), relational (child–parent agreement and parentification), behavioral (substance use and externalizing symptoms), academic (grades and self-efficacy), cultural (acculturation and bi-acculturation), and parental (parenting behaviors and parental depression). Within these dimensions, the reviewed work conceptualizes language brokers as social actors navigating complex sets of cultural and institutional norms, which often are as novel to them as they are to their parents. As they unpack contextual requirements, children cultivate a host of social, linguistic, and cognitive meta-skills. Positive experiences engender feelings of confidence and pride (DeMent & Buriel, 1999), develop linguistic and metalinguistic mastery (Malakoff & Hakuta, 1991; Valdéz, 2003), and may sharpen problem solving and varied academics skills (Kim et al., 2020; Orellana et al., 2003; Valdés, 2003). Guadalupe Valdés (2003) even associates the act with the notion of giftedness. It is also a road toward developing a sense of morality, self-efficacy, and interculturality (García-Sánchez & Orellana, 2022).

LB experiences do not always fruit positive outcomes. The practice sometimes is linked to premature adultification and stress, creating tension and resentment between children and parents. It may also interfere with time for school, friends, and personal care (Hall & Robinson, 1999; Umana-Taylor, 2003; Valenzuela, 1999; Weisskirch, 2006). Additionally, when lacking the required knowledge, children may internalize feelings of embarrassment and frustration, even inferiority (Cohen et al., 1999; Dorner et al., 2008). The pressure to know and assimilate into the new culture is also registered as a negative outcome associated with the frequency of brokering (Oznobishin & Kurman, 2017). However, the pressure of engaging in the dominant culture through LB activities can be optimized toward self-determination if children receive positive encouragement and support (Hua & Costigan, 2017).

Emerging adults and adult language brokers may participate more confidently. Ethnic identity is often realized strongly among this group, with a higher sense of responsibility and autonomy (Weisskirch, 2006, 2018). Through language brokering, young adults may nurse a deep sense of obligation toward improving family conditions and protecting family members from dominant stereotypes (Crafter & Iqbal, 2020; Reynolds & Orellana, 2009). They may also inspire parents to reclaim their pre-immigration status (Guan et al., 2016; Nash, 2017).

From the parents' perspective, dependency on family members provides a comfortable and convenient choice. Katz (2014b) notes that parents perceive ad hoc translators as unfriendly and inaccessible, acting rushed when called out of their regular duties to help with translation. Milagro, a participant in Katz's study, reflects on soliciting the help of ad hoc interprets in doctors' offices where she brokers regularly for her father:

> You have some Spanish speakers there, but sometimes the receptionists are not having a good day, and it is understandable, but . . . they're not that polite. And I've noticed that a lot . . . they'll try to rush through things, and just try to get through as fast as they can . . . and that is the thing about my dad; he feels bad and he has to go through that, and you know he prefers for me to go over there (Katz, 2014b, p. 83).

Milagro is able to read her father's discomfort when having to rely on strangers who appear bothered by answering translation requests unexpectedly. For the same reason, a thirteen-year-old girl, who regularly accompanies her mother to a Women, Infants, Children office (WIC), shares, "My mom is more comfortable having me there to explain things the right way, even though many of the staff members spoke Spanish" (Katz, 2014, p. 83). Depending on family members provides a sense of familiarity and control over unintelligible situations as well as a sense of protection when maneuvering around unknown grounds. Sometimes, both children and parents use LB as an opportunity to socialize in each other's familiar domain; the children socialize their parents in the dominant language and culture, while the parents socialize their children in the heritage language and culture (García-Sánchez, 2010; Nash, 2017).

Nonetheless, this dichotomic consideration of the LB practice in terms of good versus bad outcomes is somewhat unrealistic in representing the realities of children's translation. Recent studies have adopted wider perspectives to understand how children of all ages balance the demands of managing familial expectations and the dominant societal norms. Regardless of the setting, language brokering is in essence a social and cognitive act that involves dependent and interdependent complicated processes and attitudes.

Interactional and ethnographical frameworks present LB as an ecological environment. Orellana (2009) emphasizes that both parents and children use their available linguistic repertoires as toolkits to solve tasks at hand. Eksner and Orellana (2012) exemplify how parents work cooperatively with their children to actuate meaning-making by providing words' meaning, grammatical instructions, and background information. Katz (2014b) and García-Sánchez (2014) also note that children and parents work together to reach suitable decisions by negotiating information and family needs. Through these collaborative efforts, language brokers and parents develop competencies and influence each other's lives.

This book discusses LB practices among Iraqi patients, part of the larger Arab American LB experience, which will be briefed next.

The Arabic Experience

Studies found that the LB practice among Arabic-speaking communities is visibly characterized by the sociopolitical contexts and negative ideologies associated with Arabs and Muslims in the West. In public, language brokers activate transcultural and problem-solving skills to deal with subtle and direct acts of discrimination and stereotypes toward their families and communities. Nash (2017) explores the practice of four college students from Palestine, Iraq, and Lebanon. The Palestinian language broker talked about translating a school conference between her parents and the principal to discuss an incident in which her teacher called her a child bride and submissive for wearing the hijab. Despite the damaging experience, she recalled translating the intense interaction carefully and selectively to protect her parents from feeling targeted and rejected in their community and from worrying about her when she is at school.

Nonetheless, not all experiences are negative. Some studies report positive outcomes associated with the practice, such as enhancing family values (García-Sánchez, 2014), learning the heritage language (Guan et al., 2016), and building strong bonds among family members (Nash, 2017). Among Moroccan families in Spain, García-Sánchez (2014) suggests that children's translation is viewed by both children and parents as a necessary act of managing family situations and developing cultural values in the diaspora. Nash (2017) finds education to hold a salient value among members of this community, expressed by children encouraging parents to learn the dominant language and culture so they may regain pre-immigration careers, and parents pushing their children to learn Arabic proficiently to interact comfortably in these interactions. Positive academic outcomes linked with LB are also realized among families with small children. For example, a study reported on the LB experience of three Sudanese families in Michigan who recognize the skills the children gain when translating varied media and real-life interactions (Perry & Moses, 2011).

Part of the LB dynamics in the Arabic-speaking communities reflects the nature of the Arabic language. Arabic is a diglossic language with two or more daily coexisting linguistic forms. This discursive quotidian communicational pattern is less practiced in the diaspora. Children gradually engage more with the dominant language through education, work, entertainment, friends, and other contexts. They may retain home-dialect skills but often grow up lacking formal literacy skills in their heritage language. When language brokering takes place in institutional contexts, parents and children engage in reciprocal brokering by exchanging hybrid language expertise to achieve meaning-making (Nash, 2017). Another study on Iraqi Christian families in Illinois suggests that age and gender matter when selecting the family-designated language broker (Villanueva, 2012). The study reports that girls more than boys and the oldest more than younger children often take on the responsibility of translating for parents. Some of the parents in the study were found to be U.S.-born citizens or have lived in the United States for a considerable time, albeit still soliciting their children's help.

A recent study from Sweden reveals some of the reasons behind parents' preference for family brokering over professional translation (Hadziabdic & Hjelm, 2014). Families are concerned with issues related to cultural values, such as *ḥarām* (religiously forbidden actions), embarrassment, and confidentiality. As a small community, participants express worries about the potentiality of disclosing medical and private family matters; thus, they are more inclined to rely on their bilingual children and relatives. These diverse profiles indicate the complexity of immigrants' acculturation processes.

BROKERING MEDICAL INTERACTION

The sensitivity of translating medical interactions obligates keen theoretical and empirical examinations of this context, for it underscores serious consequences for all parties involved. The absence of interpretation or the presence of errored translation could be catastrophic. In one incident, the wrong translation of one word caused a mother signing off the custody of her two children. The mother arrived at the hospital seeking medical care for her two-year-old child who had fallen off his bike and hit his head. The provider misunderstood hitting the head during the accident as hitting by abuse and therefore reported the case to the Department of Social Services, whose representatives also arrived without a translator (Flores, 2006).

The harrowing consequences if a doctor receives the wrong names of illnesses or body parts are not hard to imagine. Cohen et al. (1999) report a case of a child translating his mother's complaint by naming the stomach as the source of her pain while the mother was pointing at her throat. The situation was saved only by the doctor's attention to the mother's gestures.

The possibilities of exposing children to sensitive and critical conditions about their parents or loved ones surface as a primary concern behind the reluctance of healthcare providers to involve children in translating medical visits. In the example below, a doctor feels powerless when relaying serious news of breast cancer to a patient through her child,

> I had to use her son to say the word "cancer" to her and she was horrified and in tears, and it was just a long, messy afternoon. . . . I think he really didn't want to be in that position, because it was like him telling the bad news, not me telling the bad news. (Katz, 2014, p. 79)

Even when the situation is not as serious, children's limited linguistic or cultural knowledge might frustrate the doctors and challenge their professional competence:

> I don't want a free-flowing discussion. I ask specific questions, and I'm looking for specific answers. . . . I am following a structure in my mind that I want to complete. It's not like we're sitting down and talking about how you feel. There is a structure in my mind, and I want to complete it so that I can get an idea as to what is wrong with the child (Katz, 2014a, p. 203).

In these words, a participant in Vikki Katz's study utters what researchers have described as the biomedical concerns versus the life concerns that said to be religiously followed by physicians when collecting information about patients' cases.

The environment for translating medical materials varies widely. Family members who interpret medical visits also perform other medical-related translations, such as scheduling appointments, making and responding to phone calls from providers and pharmacies, filling medical forms, calling for ambulances, searching for medical insurance, reading medical instructions and labels, and others. These interpreting actions are emotionally loaded encounters and have vital impacts on health conditions in ways no less important than the medical visit itself. Although they are commonly listed as part of what children do to help their relatives with health-related translations, limited knowledge is available on the dynamics and difficulties by which these interactional vignettes are managed.

A couple of recent studies stand as an anomaly to fill this gap with insightful views. Through a focus-group study design, Martinez et al. (2017)

examine the children's translation in health-insurance settings. Only three out of seventeen students from a high school in Los Angeles reported a direct involvement with translating health-insurance materials and interactions, albeit all participants indicated listening and learning from family discussions on the matter. More importantly, the study notes an active parent's role demonstrated by a strong hold on issues related to the family healthcare. Children report that their mothers overcome the language barrier and gather information independently by talking to friends and neighbors and deciding accordingly on health-insurance policies.

Many families prefer to depend on their children because of the children's abilities to understand and read their parents' emotions, as beautifully stated by a mother about her fourteen-year-old language broker: "Those people there may speak my language, but my daughter speaks my heart" (Katz, 2014b, p. 83). Children may also play a diplomatic role to ensure civil engagement. The same study describes an interesting experience of the language broker, Aurora. Aurora's parents learned that their health insurance was dormant, so they directed their frustration toward the office staff and doctors. Through translation, Aurora subtly changes their anger to a diplomatic talk by putting the blame on the insurance company, not the office staff. As a result of Aurora's approach, the office manager took on the responsibility of solving the problem. Sampling these incidents shows that we cannot underestimate the difficult positioning of children in the context of medical brokering.

Our knowledge about how language barriers affect healthcare issues in our diverse immigrant populations is considerably limited. The doctor–patient interaction, whether translated by family members or professionally, is a suitable analytical ground to produce knowledge on the topic. In this section, we will review some groundbreaking studies that have opened the doors into this site that affects the general healthcare system as much as it affects immigrant families.

There is a scarcity of research on LB in healthcare contexts for many reasons, some of which may underly the international shortage of providing interpreting services. Layperson translation in institutional settings is increasingly regulated in the United States and Europe. Hospitals and clinics are obligated under federal laws to provide language support for limited-English-speaking patients (Angelelli, 2004). In August 2000, President Bill Clinton signed Executive Order 13166 into law which obligates federal governments to be multilingual by providing oral and written multilingual support in the state's organized and funded institutions. However, studies continue to report on the limited availability of interpreters in popular as well as uncommon languages. The general attitude of policymakers and directors is "we want to stop them" (Katz, 2014b, p. 80), not recognizing or admitting that children's presence in the healthcare system is partly due to lacking appropriate institutional accommodations.

In California, AB 292 in 2003 and 2004 tried to pass a law to prevent child brokering in medical healthcare settings. Although the bill did not pass, many NGOs, hospitals, and clinics work to constrain children's translation in healthcare settings. Sometimes, to avoid the risk of being perceived as insensitive to patients' wishes, healthcare staff may leave LB unacknowledged when occurring randomly without the ability to control it. Regardless of prohibiting policies and the availability of professional support, language brokering continues to be a common strategy for managing the healthcare system among immigrant families. Katz (2014a&b) confirms that all children in her studies report interpreting medical visits and all physicians she interviewed claim frequent engagement with child brokers. Many reasons support the continuity of child brokering in medical contexts, such as convenience, trust, cultural values, socioeconomic status, and immigration status. Still, caring for family members remains as a strong motivator for the commonality of family interpretation, as articulated below by a sixteen-year-old girl from Bangladesh:

> They will arrange someone for you, but we don't do that basically, 'cause we go with her [mother]. It's easier for her, for her to explain to us than to the other person, 'cause they don't know what they, how they are going to translate and things like that, and we know her and how she is feeling and things like that so we could translate easier for her. That's it basically. (Free et al., 2003, p. 531)

Sometimes, emerging adults and adult brokers who are aware of the widespread negative ideologies surrounding certain cultural artifacts and values insist on accompanying their parents to ensure proper contact and to support their general well-being, as it appears in the intensity by which this college-age Arab language broker talks about her experiences:

> Sometimes, even if my mom doesn't ask, I go with her. Sometimes, I even skip my classes, not very often, but sometimes, I do. I mostly tell her my time so she knows when to make her appointments. I went to all her interviews. That is very important because it's not just to improve her health, but also to improve her medical support. Sometimes they do not let me translate for her because they want professional translators, but I still go with her and explain to her everything after. (Nash, 2017, p. 121)

As articulated above, families coordinate their times and efforts to support parents' health even when strict rules against family interpretation are instilled. The young interpreter above, Huda from Iraq, accompanies her mother to ensure proper treatments:

> Sometimes when they measure her blood pressure, they just remove her sleeves and they order her without being nice to her, and I am like, "Be nice to her." And when they see me understand English, they say, "Sorry, we're in a hurry." And they become nice. . . . I think it is because my mom is wearing a head covering and she does not speak English they do not treat her well. They can't take advantage of my mom just because she dresses differently or she does not speak English. I can be aggressive because I want them to be nice to my parents. I want things to be right for my parents. (Nash, 2017, p. 126)

It is expected in the medical domain that nurses and doctors are privileged to handle patients' bodies in ways that are not allowed to other strangers, but the professionalism of the healthcare marketplace normalizes and regulates this contextually required behavior through rules, such as informing the patient prior to or while operating on their bodies. The language barrier must not annihilate this ethical rule. The subtle act of not informing the patient before touching her body, as in the above example, could have been left unnoticed if it was not clearly confronted by the daughter as an improper, even hostile, action. In this context, the language broker is "positioned not only to hear and respond to such comments [behaviors in this case] but also to navigate these environments for their parents" (Orellana, 2009, p. 71), as articulated clearly: "I want things to be right for my parents." On such occasions, family brokers may address familial and cultural values more appropriately than professional strangers, as below:

> The Iraqi people are really scared, frightened of doctors in general, they are just like "Oh my God, maybe I have cancer." It's like the first thing they think about. I mean the doctor would say, "May you have this or that, all right, it's not a big deal." The Arabs, and especially Iraqis, are so afraid. . . . So, when the doctor says something, I would start by saying, "It's not that serious and the doctor didn't say that, but I just have to because if I don't and translate directly, they would be misunderstood." (Nash, 2017, p. 120)

The above fragment illuminates that the presence of family brokers in medical contexts is not a clear-cut issue. Surely there are risks involved, but as "language brokers standing literally and figuratively 'in the middle' between cultural worlds" (Orellana, 2009, p. 20), they may ameliorate differences productively. Although professional interpreters may be able to provide similar services, as they often come from similar cultural backgrounds, family brokers provide familiarity, emotional support, and patient advocacy. Additionally, language brokers accomplish things for doctors, nurses, and receptionists, and in doing so, they affect the institutional system substantially. Their work and services may be recognized as a position of power, as expressed by an eighteen-year-old college student, Luz, who serves as "la mano derecha" for her parents since childhood:

> I used to have to translate for my mom at the doctor's office so much that it came to the point where the doctor would only talk to me. He wouldn't even look at my mom. Instead, he would ask me for updates and symptoms. Afterward, he would give me his recommendations and had me choose what the best options would be for my mom. Often, I had to interrupt him to explain what had been going on with my mom and to ask her what she thought, but I must admit that sometimes I made choices for her without asking her first. (Orellana, 2009, p. 74)

The above fragment conveys a critical aspect of mediated encounters. The healthcare provider elects to interact with the daughter through the shared language rather than treating his patient as his first interlocutor, as revealed clearly: "he wouldn't even look at her." Through verbal and nonverbal communicational cues, the doctor positions the daughter as the decision-maker of the meeting. In that vein, he orients toward mutual intelligibility more than the social membership category that identifies the patient between his two interlocutors.

The above-discussed studies consider the language broker's side as a locus for understanding the dynamics of language brokering, but the patient's side has largely been left unexplored. In Erving Goffman's terms (1981), the patient has been treated as a *non-person*, whose presence is left to be self-determined. I hypothesize that patients may enter into the conversation on their account, not solely based on discursive institutional and interpreting expectations. This hypothesis is the angle by which the alignment and misalignment among LB participants will be noted.

Nuts and Bolts of Brokering Medical Encounters

The scenario mentioned above with the daughter being summoned as the decision-maker is certainly not a dominant LB profile in medical encounters. Sometimes, language brokers feel invisible, unsure of their position among adults, as articulated below by a sixteen-year-old boy brokering a GE visit for his mother:

> I don't know, it's sort of like when they are talking, if I and my mum are sort of like sitting next to each other and they knew we had come for my mum, they would be like talking to my mum and talking to her face and I would answer them but they would still carry on looking at my mum when they are talking, even though they know my mum can't understand. Um, sometimes it is really

> annoying because it's like I am here to help her, and you are like, you are not like looking at me sort of thing, so sometimes I don't even know if like they even listen to anything I am saying and it's like sometimes I don't think they even want me to be there . . . but I have no choice but to be there. (Free et al. 2003, p. 533)

The child broker above finds himself in the middle mediating a sensitive ground, while the doctor's facial expression and body position made him feel unwanted. This fragment points to the importance of paying attention to nonverbal cues when inferring meaning in crosslinguistic communications.

Recently, a much needed work has reviewed the field development and revealed the overwhelming shortage of LB medical research (de Abreu & O'Dell, 2017). From 1999 to 2014, only six articles focused specifically on medical contexts, whereas eight papers included medical visits as part of the general analyzed language brokering experiences, and fifty-five papers mentioned medical brokering in passing. The fourteen studies that dealt with medical brokering centered on the language broker's experiences, but two discussed the perspectives of healthcare providers (Cohen et al., 1999; Katz, 2014a & b), and three included the parents' accounts (Corona et al., 2012; Katz, 2014a & b; García-Sánchez, 2010). The review suggests that ten to seventeen years old are the most common ages of the child broker in healthcare contexts, while a five-year-old interpreting a GE visit for his mother is the youngest reported case of children's translation. The combined perspectives from the review project reveal that although the limited availability of professional interpretation services contributes to the presence of child brokers in medical contexts, parents' preferences, socioeconomic situations, and immigration status are primary reasons behind the prevalence of child brokering.

There are no comprehensive national studies that inform on the state of patients using professional versus family interpretation, but we know that the situation varies by geographical areas. De Abreu and O'Dell (2017) note that 26 percent of Spanish-speaking patients in emergency rooms need interpreters, but 22 percent of these situations were conducted without one. Patients who do not receive interpretation remain unaware of their diagnosis and unsatisfied with their medical experiences. In these situations, doctors may prefer to deal with family brokers over interacting without translation.

From the professional perspective, child brokering may threaten doctors' identities and cultural competencies. Doctors may feel unprepared to deal with different cultural values around defining the notions of childhood and privacy. Because familiar social norms are constructed in the form of adults speaking on behalf of children, the medical staff may view the practice as an invasive act that violates children's innocence and jeopardizes parents' authority. In such perspectives, parents are viewed passively, as powerlessly waiting for their children to take care of the situation, leading to a stance that contributes to internalizing biases and hindering effective communications. Some doctors are adamant about the unsuitability of children's translation, as demonstrated in a statement cited by Cohen et al. (1999, p. 166): "Under no circumstances should children be asked to interpret medical details for their parents. It appears to us to be unethical, unprofessional, uncivilized, and totally unacceptable" (Rack, 1982, pp. 199–200).

The opposing attitude about child brokering is usually based on morals and personal ethics rather than empirical proofs. Doctors are not informed by the robust statistical or qualitative data on the state of family brokering in ways that prepare them to handle these situations more effectively and positively. The situation may frustrate some doctors leading them to adopt defensive attitudes and alternative strategies, as revealed by the pediatrician below:

> I am sort of guilty for being—having like prejudged notion when I walk into a room. It's a pain that they don't speak English. . . . So it sort of centers on the kid. . . . The problem when it comes to medical translation is that they don't know the words. . . . So that when I sometimes have to pull someone from here to translate; and because they are not professional either, there are things that I'll say that, you know, they don't understand either. So I have actually a little Spanish-English dictionary that I'll use to help. (Katz, 2014a, p. 202)

The doctor above lists a number of strategies she has learned from dealing with limited-English-speaking patients, but none of which includes soliciting patients' help or observing the collaborative mother–child, verbal and nonverbal communicational cues. Sometimes, doctors may be frustrated with lacking the level of linguistic sophistication required for dealing with serious materials such as medical information, as expressed in this statement: "It is one thing to speak in vernacular. It's another thing not to know that it's vernacular. It's ridiculous" (Katz, 2014a, p. 78). These worries reflect the medical concern with the accuracy of information and manner of delivery, which encompass not only knowing the correct medical terms, but also familiarity with medical concepts, as articulated by this physician: "It's not just a language, but education. If I say: 'How frequently are you wheezing?' What I am trying to do is understand the nature of the severity of asthma, they don't understand that frequency means some sort of ratio" (Katz, 2014a, p. 203).

These testimonies clearly reveal the professional concern with the biomedical side of doctor–patient interactions. They show how doctors are oriented to receiving information in a precise manner that facilitates their work. They also show a focal concern with the child broker, leaving the patients' role and position in the dark.

Healthcare providers espouse child brokering with extra stress and feelings of uncertainty about passing their professional judgment to the child translator. As mentioned earlier, accuracy is a matter of a great concern among healthcare providers. The healthcare setting contains numerous branches and diseases. The demanding forms of knowledge and linguistic abilities in these varied contexts are unattainable and unfamiliar to most language brokers. The types of errors children make when relaying doctor's statements and how these errors influence patient's health are critical issues that are yet to be thoroughly examined, some anecdotal studies conducted mostly by medical practitioners have reflected on the seriousness of the matter (Baker et al., 1996; Flores et al., 2003; Flores, 2005, 2006). Flores et al. (2003) investigated the frequency and types of errors in mediating medical visits in a seven-month study. They collected and analyzed data from thirteen medical encounters, an average of two a month, interpreted by six professional interpreters, six ad hoc social and hospital workers, and one eleven-year-old sibling. The study found a high number of errors, about 31 percent per visit, common among all groups, most of which were omissions (52 percent) and false fluency (16 percent). The errors of the ad hoc interpreters have a higher potential for clinical consequences than those committed by professional interpreters (77 percent vs. 53 percent). The study discloses clearly the commonality of errors in mediated medical encounters, a truly uncomfortable situation to be left without serious examination, considering that the ad hoc interpreters in the study were bilingual hospital staff.

Yet still, some providers view language brokers' presence positively, acknowledging their work in facilitating less stressful encounters, providing extra information on the family health situation and shortening consultation time. Through these narratives and interviews, we are informed about critical aspects surrounding child brokering, but thus far, we have learned that parents may prefer to work with their children and work with them to facilitate meaning-making over soliciting the help of professional interpreters.

In that vein, the sentiments that encourage parents to rely on their bilingual relatives, motivated by perceiving non-family interpreters as unhelpful and unfriendly, are not too far from the actual situation on the ground. Nonetheless, any errored communication leading to serious health consequences is enough to motivate preventative measures, which unnecessarily should be translated into eliminating one form of interpretation for the sake of the other.

POLICIES AND REGULATIONS

Several policies attempt to regulate language disparities in healthcare settings. Title VI of the Civil Rights Act of 1964 established the need for professional interpreters. In 2000, President Clinton signed into law an order to facilitate equal access for limited-English-speaking patients. In 2008, a nationwide survey from the National Health Law Program assessed the development of language accessibility and re-established the importance of closing the gap in healthcare quality due to language barriers. By 2019, most states have issued at least three laws addressing foreign language services in healthcare settings, while California has 257 provisions, the highest number among all states. The policies were issued to obligate hospitals and clinics to provide professional interpreting services and to limit or diminish the use of child brokering.

In response to these official efforts, federal organizations and NGO have established training programs, interpreting certifications, and codes of ethical conduct (Angelelli, 2004). The general guidelines for healthcare interpretations were originally borrowed from the court and conference interpretation describing the preferred manners of transferring information between patients and doctors objectively and neutrally. In other words, the expectation is to perform interpretation without personal agency so that professionalism is defined by the level of invisible positionality. On the professional ground, however, empirical studies prove that these expectations are far from reality (Angelelli, 2004, 2014; Davidson, 2000, 2002).

The Interpreter's Story

Formal policies are not always practiced verbatim. Joseph M. Kaufert and Robert W. Putsch (1997) collected twenty codes of conduct from healthcare institutions and found them overwhelmingly emphasizing neutrality and objectivity as goals of successful professional interpreting. In contrast, examining interpreters' performance empirically reveals a wide discrepancy between how the interpreter's role is described on paper and how it is practiced on the ground. Through multiple studies, Claudia V. Angelelli asserts the interpreter's agency in shaping their realities and the realities of their customers (Angelelli, 2014).

A few elements are critical when constructing such realities. Cultures, language usage, and expectations position the interpreters in a critical place, sometimes in zones of dilemma and conflict. Despite institutional recommendations, interpreters do not perform their job as conduits but as text authors, communicational coordinators, institutional gatekeepers, or patient advocates. However, when caught in the middle, they lean toward representing the employing agency, which may contribute to the limited-English-speaking patients' disempowerment. Ultimately, professional interpreters are state-trained and certified employees, working in state-supported institutions (hospitals, clinics, and courts), and programs (colleges and vocational schools). On these accounts, professional interpreters may maintain forms of institutional asymmetries.

Taking the interpreters' perspectives on navigating the complexity of their job reveals their awareness of the sensitive ground they occupy. They feel restricted by their obligation toward their institutional training and expectations, even when they sense the need to advocate for patients. In that light, some professional interpreters understand and sympathize with patients who prefer to conduct their work with family interpreters (Fatahi et al., 2005).

From the institutional side, research paints a deficit picture of interpreters' accessibility and accuracy. Studies show that interpreting services are insufficiently available in U.S. healthcare systems and offer limited choices besides the commonly used languages. Even when available, physicians rarely call for interpreting services, finding the situation inefficient when entering the examination room and having to call for interpretation services. Lee et al. (2006) note that doctors sometimes opt to rely on their own bilingual skills or bilingual staff, or even may choose to conduct business without much interaction with their non-English-speaking patients. Even if services are available, other difficulties may hamper their effective utility. Patients must be informed about the form of available interpreting services in the facilities where they receive treatment and they must know how to request help, which also requires language and cultural skills. In these conditions, doctors may be ambivalent about the presence of the children's brokering and may even prefer it. Additionally, the practice may carry more values than deserving an abolition or uncooperative attitudes.

CONCLUSION

This book contributes to scholarly conversations in interpretive and medical research by analyzing the processes of meaning-making as actuating in different parts of brokered medical encounters. For the rest of the book, the analyzes will include the micro-verbal and nonverbal actions of three interlocutors: doctors, patients, and language brokers, with a central focus on understanding the position and actions of limited-English-speaking patients, the ways in which they conduct their speakership to handle an important aspect of their life as their health.

This chapter presents opposite views on the matter of depending on family interpreting. By reviewing these claims and the advantages and disadvantages associated with the practice of language brokering among immigrant families in medical contexts, I neither rally behind the dependency on language brokering nor against it. Instead, I concur with the belief that families' reliance on internal help in the capacity of interpretation and translation will continue regardless of regulating policies and negative research findings. From that perspective, cultivating knowledge on the practice among different immigrant communities to support patients' choice and institutional efforts is a better course of action to build a caring and responsive healthcare system.

Chapter 1

The Interaction of Medicine and Art

Key Concepts and Theoretical Applications

This chapter discusses the argument for espousing the scholarships of social sciences and medicine. It samples the growing collaboration between conversation analysis and doctor–patient interaction to examine institutionally produced and sustained behaviors. The interactional paradigm of competence in contexts of diversity and limitations will also be reviewed as a pathway into understanding how immigrant patients constitute their patienthood.

Doctors deal with several patients a day, some of their meetings are successful, and others are not. Unpacking the reasons behind such disparity is crucial when consistency and equality are the objectives of the healthcare system. A promising method of achieving this objective is examining medical interactions through the utility of recordings. The advancement of modern technology has encouraged researchers to advocate for the use of recordings in producing knowledge on medical conduct. A prominent initiative in this direction is *Doctor, His Patient, and the Illness* by Michael Balint (1957). The work reports on recordings of weekly gatherings of fourteen doctors with a psychiatrist for several years to discuss problems related to practicing medicine. The author prescribed that doctors ought to learn from failed and successful cases by recording and sharing personal experiences.

Another groundbreaking project is the *The Doctor and His Patient: A Sociological Interpretation* by Samuel W. Bloom (1963) establishes the case for espousing social sciences and medicine as an essential connection to study and improve the doctor–patient relationship. Directed at students of medicine, Bloom reminds his readers of the historical link between art and medicine, noting that reclaiming this lineage helps doctors to see their patients as more than a sum of parts and to understand their cases as human conditions rather than scientific problems. Bloom advises from a personal experience as a professor of social sciences at the College of Medicine, Baylor University

A seminal project has come to build an early case for the vitality of using recordings in studying medical conduct. Based on large data pulled from recordings of 2,500 primary-care consultations, *The Doctor Talking to Patients* (Byrne & Long, 1976) anatomizes the structure of medical visits and details several doctors' behaviors. It was the first to note that medical visits exhibit fixed timing and order of interactional phases through which meetings are forwarded according to doctors' initiatives.

The recommendations of these early precursors and the availability of recording devices have encouraged a wide surge in medical behavioral research through quantitative and qualitative studies. These developments, coinciding with the emergence of conversation analysis (CA) and ethnomethodology as fields of studying common sense and meaning-making, have provided a robust scientific ground to usher in the interactional research of medicine. Since this early advocacy, significant knowledge has been produced. Presently, the imprint of espousing social sciences and medical research is an accomplished fact, albeit it is at a state of infancy in the context of crosslinguistic encounters where gaps of understandings assert themselves.

SOCIAL MEDICAL RESEARCH

The early collaborations between social sciences and medicine were built largely on aggregation techniques, known as process analyses, that employ a coding system of large, compiled samples to examine behavioral features in terms of task-focused and socioemotional categories. These techniques have established medical communication as a valid field of observation and research with potentials to systematically improve healthcare quality. Significant knowledge was produced through the utility of the Roter Interactional Analysis System (RIAS), which consists of 39 categories, 15 emotional features, and 24 focus-task features, used especially with research in the primary-care medicine. Although RIAS has facilitated the collection of some exhaustive and other prominent features of medical interactions and has established social medical research as a valid inquiry ground into improving healthcare quality, the method was criticized for its heavy focus on extraneous variables (Heritage & Maynard, 2006). The findings of these early orientations created a solid ground for the developing methodology of studying the doctor-patient relationship through micro and internal features.

Grounded in anthropological and sociological perspectives, social research moved forward to examine medical interactions through interpretive methods, the focal attention examines the ways in which structures of power shape individuals' experiences and influence how interactions are formed and progressed (Heritage & Maynard, 2006; Giddens, 1984). Based on this orientation, most of the earlier patient–doctor social research reflects a relationship fraught with features of power asymmetries (Cicourel, 1981; Mishler, 1984; Waitzkin, 1984; West, 1983, 1984; Todd & Fisher, 1993). Mishler (1984) finds doctor–patient rapport to represent a fixed manner in the norm of doctors asking questions and patients providing answers. West (1983) notes that doctors introduce, develop, and change topics through questions as an interactional paradigm that helps in sustaining doctors' control over the encounter. Shuy (1993) suggests that patients' questions are treated as less relevant to the visit's progressivity and are often used for labeling rather than enhancing understanding. Christian Heath (1992) argues that although the asymmetry in doctor–patient relationships is institutionally structured, it is however interactionally preserved when patients choose to follow traditional patterns of communication. Finally, Paul ten Have (1991) suggests that while doctors generally control moving interactions forward, both parties contribute to asymmetrical interactional patterns if patients passively refrain from asking questions or giving comments. In summary, these early works note that if doctors' verbal and nonverbal presentations are faced with patients' silence, doctors proceed, suggesting that patient's disempowerment is constructed and sustained mutually between doctors and patients.

An anomaly to this dominant view is a pioneer work that advised for a contextual understanding of doctor-patient interactions based on the specificity of medical branches. Thomas S. Szasz and Marc H. Hollender (1956) posit that linking social behaviors with organic symptoms points to three types of doctor–patient relationships: (1) activity-passivity, (2) guidance-cooperation, and (3) mutual participation. The activity-passivity model is originated from the emergency medicine where decisions are left entirely to doctors, especially when patients are taking as being more or less helpless. The guidance-cooperation model describes a parental prototype relationship fitting mostly in domains of acute disorders, such as infectious diseases. The patient is expected to look up to the doctors' expertise and cooperate with their recommendation. The mutual participation model works with chronic-disease cases, doctors guide patients to manage their health, but ultimately patients are responsible for their well-being. In this latter model, patients are expected to be active in organizing and managing their health through the assistance of periodic consultations. These relational categories challenge the then-prevailing assumption that a general interactional behavior governs all types of medical conduct.

In reviewing these classic efforts, I certainly do not discredit their claims. Nonetheless, our increasingly complicated and super-diverse world invites us to study social interactions in the light of their internal and local environments. As noted, doctors have good and bad experiences. Beyond the judgment value, the ultimate goal of social sciences in medicine is to augment the communicational patterns leading to good experiences and eliminating those that contribute to failed meetings. A solid coda cultivated from social research is that successful and failed encounters are heavily structured by interactional factors. That is indeed encouraging. As delivered, most of bad experiences are interactionally constructed, and in that vein, they can be interactionally repaired. As hard sciences are steadily advancing, social sciences can mobilize their advancement through effective communication.

Part of the set orientations of the early work could be in effect due to the adopted field coinage. Unites of description may or may not present a problem in the examined interactional scenes, but they may impound ways of initial thinking into certain directions (Gumperz, 1981). This issue of labeling definitely has not passed unnoticed among prominent social theorists and analysists (Agar, 1975; Goodwin, 1990; Gumperz, 1981; Hymes, 1974). Gumperz, (1981) posits that, "The very labels we use are often quite different from what we really intend to do" (p. 12). In her early ethnographic work, Marjorie H. Goodwin notes that no specific names were designated to label the children's games she encountered at the Maple Street, promoting her to refrain from employing any culturally loaded lexemes in reference to these activities. Goodwin argues that "even when labels do exist, they might not provide any straightforward insight into the phenomena they name" (Goodwin, 1990, p. 23). In the context of social medical research, the embraced terms might have hegemonically directed the research field into a preset tone. For example, the term doctor-patient *conference* is unfaithfully attached to medical encounters along with the overwhelmingly employed term, doctor-patient interviews. The Oxford Dictionary (Stevenson, 2010) defines the lexeme *conference* as "an official meeting at which people with the same work or interest come together to discuss their views" (p. 12). Thus, a *conference* represents a multiparty meeting progressing on the basis of the mutual interests and contributions of its participants. Contrastively, the term *interview* denotes a formal and fixed-role interaction between an interviewer and an interviewee. The early medical behavioral research profiles unyielding interactional patterns, but later developed conversation analytical studies increasingly depict various norms as shaped and reshaped by medical domains and local contexts. Nonetheless, the social medical research has utilized the term *interview* when referencing the doctor-patient interaction much more widely than other labels. Given that the term *conference* and interview are historically loaded lexemes and bounded with distinguished interactional settings, I became rather inclined to rely on a broader label to discuss mediated medical meetings. In this book, I settled on the term, *encounter*.

Early claims on doctor-patient conduct underscore an element of consensus, which might have contributed to a widespread standpoint regarding patients' disempowerment. However, by identifying patients as culprits in sustaining power asymmetries, we ultimately contribute to their marginalization. In essence, we are identifying them as responsible for the excluding patterns that negatively shape their medical experiences. Yet, a danger, as I view it, resides in dismissing the characteristic ways of contextual specificity that shape interactions differentially. Communicational skills diversly privilege and empower patients' voice at institutional and national levels. Recent research directions have begun to shed light on social disparities and communicational asymmetries among vulnerable patients. Patients with higher education and communicational proficiencies are better heard than patients with language barriers and low health literacy (Hoffman et al. 2011). Moreover, socioeconomically vulnerable patients receive fewer positive communications, less guided mutual decision-making, and less explanation about their diagnosis (Baker et al. 1996; Cohen et al., 1999; Flores et al., 2003; Free et al., 2003; Martinez et al., 2019).

Beyond broad social structures, asymmetrical patterns should also be judged against the background of internal interactional features. Healthier perspectives may be cultivated from conceptualizing the doctor–patient relationship as an encounter between two equally and contextually essential parties so that the presence of one party actuates the identity of the other, as an individual with an illness account seeking advice from an expert. Studying the inner mobilizing details of doctor–patient interactions elucidates such understandings, the features of which can be delineated through educational and training programs.

The Developing Field of Interactional Medical Research

The onset of the CA medical research perhaps can be pinned down to Harvey Sacks' lectures between the Fall of 1964 and Spring of 1965 at the University of California in Irvine and the University of Los Angeles. He started by analyzing the transcripts of three recorded phone calls to an emergency psychiatric hospital, and he systematically explained how callers may provide or counsel their identities in response to the opening questions of phone conversations with staff members (Sacks, 1992). These analyses became the basis for studying the rules of conversational sequencing, a line of research developed from Sack's early work with Harold Garfinkel and Erving Goffman. His collaboration with Emanuel Schegloff and Gail Jefferson in the 1970s is pronounced by most as the birth of CA research. By the time Sacks died in 1975, CA was established as a robust scientific and analytical approach for studying problems of communication in institutional and casual settings.

Western medicine is increasingly moving toward patient-centered healthcare. Informing and involving patients may balance the power relationship immanent in the exchange between life knowledge and biomedical knowledge that marks doctor–patient interactions with features of asymmetries.

The method by which information is gathered to examine this relationship vitally influences how knowledge is produced and disseminated. CA has addressed issues related to the overall structure of medical encounters and the micro-details of how intersubjectivity is achieved and construed. One of the key achievements of CA approaches is studying the sequential organization of interactions based on a few primary operational princ:pals, mainly that all social interactions have an internal and systematic structure, all verbal and non-verbal actions are potentially related and meaningful to the ongoing interaction, and all these actions are context-shaped and context-renewing.

Through these three basic assumptions, studying social interactions through CA approaches can be optimized by one or a combination of the following four components:

1. The overall structure of interactions
2. The sequence of turn-taking
3. A single-turn design
4. A specific lexicon

The overall structure of social interaction may illuminate the distribution of talk through incorporating language forms with social structures. For example, the social interaction of the medical visit contains six stages: opening and problem presentations, history taking, physical examination, diagnosis, treatment plans, and closing (Byrne & Long, 1976). By employing CA paradigms, some aspects of these phases have been identified (Halkowski, 2006; Heritage & Robinson, 2006; Heritage & Maynard, 2006; Maynard & Heritage, 2005). The opening of the medical visit provides an institutionally built space for disclosing patients' concerns (Heritage & Robinson, 2006); the history-taking phase is organized to embody physicians' understanding of the medical problem (Boyd & Heritage, 2006), while most decision and diagnosis phases are treated strictly as a medical-domain space where doctors give their expert opinions. Despite such institutionally-built structures, patients may resist hegemonical patterns to advance their agendas based on their agency. For example, patients' concerns are institutionally localized in the visits' opening, but patients are found to continue revealing their concerns throughout the visit, usually in narrative forms.

Concerning inner- and micro-features of medical interactions, a primary focus is on understanding the forces that motivate and shape the doctor–patient rapport. For example, Douglas W. Maynard (1997) examines how diagnostic talks are delivered as good versus bad news. Wayne A. Beach (1993, 1995, 2020) notes the functions of small talk—such as *okay*—in a series of studies in oncology and primary-care visits. Tanya Stivers (2005b, 2006) shows how patients fashion their responses in ways that predict their cooperation with or rejection of the treatment plan, while Heritage and McArthur (2019) demonstrate how the orientation of doctors' gaze encourage patients' cooperation and satisfaction.

The manner of delivering medical opinions captures wide interest among CA researchers. In acute visits, Heritage and Stivers (1999) categorize medical decisions into three types: pre-diagnosis, online commentary, and diagnosis. The authors distinguish the online-commentary statements to show how doctors use certain formula of decision delivery to communicate mild conditions and absences of problems, asserting that such forms never appeared with serious problems in all their collected data. These statements come in the form of "I don't see any problem" or "that feels normal," often verbalized during the examination stage to downgrade patients' evaluations and worries.

While previous work claimed general patients' passive behavior, CA studies have shown that patients' attitudes and actions might vary by medical domains. Stivers (2005b) finds that prescribing antibiotics in acute pediatric care is only reached by achieving an accord between doctors and mothers. Wayne Beach and Erin Prickett (2017) note that patients use laughter when facing challenging circumstances with their cancer conditions, an action that is not shared nor reciprocated by doctors. While social studies generally show the influence of certain social variables such as age, gender, and education, on patterns of participation, CA studies increasingly focus on producing knowledge on the doctor-patient rapport by specifying features of interactions as related to local contexts of the medical domain or stage.

As a means of collecting information to support medical hypotheses, question designs have received wide attention among CA scholars. John Heritage (2010) points out that medical questions are not formed in ordinary styles as survey and other fixed type instruments. For example, a question about marital status is solicited in a form that requires a simple yes/no answer, such as "Are you married?" and "Are you divorced?" while a survey-type question is formed neutrally in an objective manner similar to "What is your marital status?" These questions are designed in a way to cast some control over the direction of the interaction, but also to serve doctor-patient rapport. Doctors are instructed by formal rules and training to develop rapport with their patients as a primary function of the medical interviews to serve gathering information about the medical problem, educating patients about their illness, and motivating patients to adhere to treatment plans (Cohen-Cole, 1991). Heritage shows that doctors form their questions in a way that predicts the best-scenario response and allows a confirmation of "the best guess," as in the example below.

(Heritage, 2010, p. 15):

DOC: Is it? what-w: it's just milk coming up, no: 'hhh
No blood or anyt'ing gree[n or anything ¿
CLR: [No:,

The doctor's question above is designed in a way that communicates a strong preference for a certain response. It also suggests the valence of expectation through which the epistemological stance of the doctor or the patient is confirmed (Heritage, 2010, 2012). Heritage also notes that doctors navigate the question design in ways that show how they may set a side their medical agenda to respond to patients' lifestyle inputs.

The functions of agenda setting in forming doctors' questions are also examined by Jeffery Robinson (2006). Robinson demonstrates that doctors form their questions in ways that communicate their understanding of whether the patient's case is new, follow-up, or chronicle. New-concern questions are often designed in some form of "What can I do for you today?" or "How can I help you today?" and other types of open-ended questions. While a question such as "How do you feel today?" is designed to solicit an answer about a follow-up visit. Patients respond in a manner that communicates their orientation to the doctor's question design and doctors' understanding of their cases. These exemplary works feature one of the foundational achievements of the CA paradigm, namely marking the relevancy between interactional turns at talk as analytically visible (Goodwin, 1979; Heritage, 1984; Sacks & Schegloff, 1979; Schegloff, 1991).

The increasing number of reviews that attempt to synthesize research findings, populations, and objectives is a valid indicator of the growth of CA medical research. Beach and colleagues (2017) sum the findings of ten review articles to show field achievements from 1997 to 2015. Their review strongly builds the case for combining qualitative and quantitative analyses to improve healthcare quality and training programs, robustly demonstrating how CA methodology has sufficient and operative built-in tools to examine the values and currency of interactional features in a single case, a limited number of cases, and a large data set.

CA researchers continue to unpack details of the power relationship between doctors and patients, such as the environments that trigger or suppress collaborative meaning-making; therefore, the local operative forces behind effective or failed outcomes may be procedurally discerned (Maynard & Heritage, 2005). The claim that CA approaches promise to offer effective measures in reaching quality healthcare has gained support by Heritage and associates' work (2007) by showing how unmet patients' concerns are reduced by 75 percent when doctors receive training based on CA methodologies and findings.

INTERACTIONAL COMPETENCE

Studying interactional competence is ultimately a study into the geography of social cognition—a study of the human faculty that allows building contextually appropriate actions (Clark, 1985; Edwards, 2006). In groundbreaking works, Charles Goodwin (1943–2018) demonstrates the ways in which relevant actions can elucidate interactional competencies through the employment of simultaneously organized semiotic resources. Goodwin argues that only by expanding the analysis beyond grammatical abilities of individuals to encompass sequencing of talk and embodied action "that we can theorize about human ability" (Goodwin, 2004, p. 151).

To support the veracity of his conceptual offering behind the pragmatism of cognition, Goodwin analyzes the actions of Chil, an aphasic patient whose stroke left him with no more than three words—and, yes, and no. He demonstrates how Chil's linguistic repertoire, though limited, creates the environments that allow Chil to embed himself as an effective partner in conversations. By latching to interlocutor's prior talk, Chil builds complex actions, such as adding, listing, contradicting, and evaluating (Goodwin, 2004, 2013). Chil's pragmatic abilities are rendered visible and meaningful only when considering the semiotic resources in his environment upon which he builds his actions relevantly (Goodwin, 2000; Goodwin & Goodwin, 2004). Primacy among those resources is the simple yet powerful enactment of human cognition through monitoring the ongoing interactions.

The act of monitoring interactional details allows Chil to perform and operate on complicated action. Relying on prosody and gesture, he displays an affect, enacts a stance, and constructs a list so that he is perceived and treated as a speaker with relevant contributions to the group's collective interactional goal. Crucial is to note that the relevant attention field is mutually constituted among Chil and his conversationalists as an environmentally necessary axiom to facilitate the progressivity of meaning-making. Through such a pragmatic enactment of attention, actions become the context for the next action. For example, Chil produces a string of what can be considered nonsense, "Nih nih duh duh Da duh" (Goodwin, 2018, p. 61). However, this string of utterances actuates the relatedness and provides conditions for forming the recipient's turn. For example, Chil uses similar tunic items to an act "duh dih Da" and another, "no no no," to perform varied actions, such as listing and assessments. These three verbalization-type expressions are delivered in different tunes and successfully achieve a range of actions. Chil's actions underscore profound cognitive and contextual abilities mobilized by the following resources: (1) the effective utility of micro-interactional contexts—building turns by operating on prior turns, (2) an excellent, yet not perfect, perception—a pragmatic enactment of intention, (3) things in the environment—his seat and body orientation, participants' field of attention, and finally (4) the sentiment of caring—the guiding effort to building mutual understandings (see figure 1.1).

Goodwin's theoretical and empirical paradigm of analyzing human's cognition and sociability is indispensably linked to the context of interaction, with the term *context* referring to both the local environment of an utterance and the background of a given interaction (Duranti & Goodwin, 1992). It is a framework built to render interactional competence contextually relevant, and on this basis, it is best examined in challenging environments. Research studies on interactions of non-native speakers' (Firth, 1990; Wagner & Firth, 1997), infant verbalization (Lee et al., 2009), communication of autistic children (Ochs & Solomon, 2010), and interactions in bilingual classrooms (Seedhouse, 2004) are examples of analyzing contexts marked with linguistic, cognitive, and cultural diversity.

In this study, I adopted Goodwin's framework to study patterns of participation and speakership in brokered medical encounters. Certainly, there is an obvious and profound difference between the two contexts. Language brokering (LB) participants have a wider range of linguistic repertoire at their disposal, much more complicated than what is available in Chil's case.

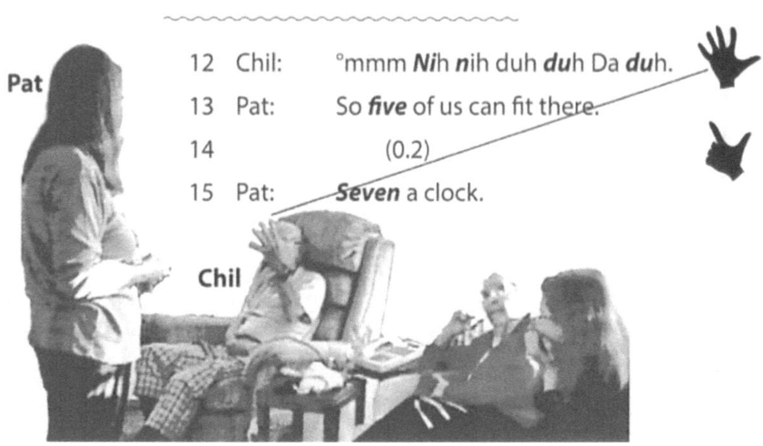

Figure 1.1 The Decomposition of Prior Talk. Credit: Cambridge University Press. Used with permission.

However, the study draws impetus from the conceptual paradigm through which Goodwin builds indisputable evidence that mutual linguistic intelligibility is by no means the only way in which people enact their communicative competence.

CA and interactional competence are the analytical frameworks I employ to study the actions of limited-English-speaking patients. From its inception, CA was developed to examine the sequential organization of interactional turns. The CA paradigm started as a sociological project, and developed to offer profound psychological underpinnings, as carried and enhanced by Goodwin's method of rendering the cognitive zone of attention analytically visible, robustly so in challenging environments. This empirical display of the theoretical understanding of the geography of cognition that underscores the CA paradigm addresses a vital element that hard sciences have worked diligently to prove, namely the neural plasticity. Interactionally, Goodwin and associates demonstrate that the human mind is mart with abilities that are not fixed, fossilized, or predetermined. Human mind is a zone of rebirthing and re-wiring associative connections between, social, linguistic, and cognitive elements.

CROSSLINGUISTIC MEDICAL ENCOUNTERS

The scholarships on same-language medical conduct offers insightful perspectives to study crosslinguistic medical interactions. Since immigrant patients with limited-English skills communicate in institutional settings built and run by English speakers their interactions are also subjected to institutional features of same-language medical encounters. On these bases, I hypothesize that participatory norms of limited-English-speaking patients are shaped by at least five internal and external elements:

1. The language broker's bilingual abilities
2. The language broker's sense of responsibility
3. The medical institutional norms
4. The doctor's orientation toward the brokering dynamics
5. The patient's agency

Unpacking these elements is the endeavor of this project with a central objective to understand the positionality of limited-English-speaking patients, through which they exercise a complicated set of cognitive and interactional competencies.

CONCLUSION

Before moving forward to engage with brokered medical encounters, backing our discussions with the knowledge produced on same-language doctor-patient conduct became vital, which was the basic dedication of this chapter. The succinct review provided here is by no means an exhaustive project. Rather, it is an entrance into the growing field of social medical research guided by an objective to situate the present work within studies that enlightened some of the complexities of medical conducts as a primordial for social interactions. This project interacts with related scholarships on medical interactions, language brokering, and interactional competency. It focuses on examining the roles through which patients manage to engage in their medial interactions.

Doctors usually do not receive special training when working with underserved communities and vulnerable patients; the general medical training and education are the resources by which they conduct their professionalism toward patients from all flex of cultural and linguistic backgrounds. Some doctors may accumulate valuable experiences because of the geographical areas where they work, but these experiences are structured according to personal processes, dispositions, and biases rather than rigorous scientific evidence. I hope this work will encourage future pathways into building a corpus of data to support medical teams successfully and confidently when working with patients from diverse linguistic and cultural backgrounds. Such an orientation allows us to view diversity as a context for enriching the art of medicine.

Chapter 2

Ethnographic Notes

The Poetics of Collecting Language-Brokering Vignettes

This chapter narrates the trajectory of this project. It discusses the design of the study and provides information about the nuts and bolts of collecting real-life vignettes of language brokering. Thus, its main purpose is to describe the site where data was collected, participating families, the language of the researched community, and the method of analysis. It concludes by discussing with my readers a few thoughts related to research methodologies.

Collecting data of naturally occurring multiparty interactions is a challenging task on many fronts. A researcher must navigate several sensitive issues when collecting audio and videos of real-time interactions. Sometimes, the difficulties are purely technical, such as preparing the right equipment suitable for different sites, angles, and events, and other times, unexpected events may interfere with the process. As we ask people to act as naturally as possible, they may move around or change their seating arrangement so that they fall outside the camera frame when their actions are still relevant to the investigated phenomena. In an incident, while recording a child translating a TV show for his mother, their neighbor stopped by and was invited over for tea. I certainly had to terminate the recording, since the visitor was an unconsented participant. More importantly, collecting data of people managing their daily lives is a sensitive endeavor for the researcher as much as it is for the families. It is a delicate negotiation of cultural values and personal traits that ought to be grounded in a profound sense of responsibility and humanity. Even the field-designated vocabulary items, such as *data* or *subject*, are uncomfortable to use when referring to real-life moments of family members discussing aspects of their lives.

These processes ease considerably when relationships are built before the fieldwork. During all parts of the study, researchers must inform participants about their rights and the options available to them. They should be confidently aware of all details culminating in the completion of their involvement with the study, including choosing the start and the end of their participation. For example, they may decide where and when data can be collected (e.g., which visit, which doctor). Sometimes, families offer to share a meal or a drink before work; these incidents must be gracefully honored to build a trusting relationship. Other families may decide to keep their engagement strictly formal, preferring, for example, to meet at the place of the data recording to limit family exposure; these demands surely must be granted. In the context of language brokering, many families are recent immigrants and may need help with directions, transportation, and communication. Depending on the families' preference and the study design, researchers should not shy away from assisting when needed.

DATA OF BROKERING MEDICAL ENCOUNTERS

Due to the nature of language brokering—an activity of oral and written translation occurring on demand among friends and family members—capturing examples on videos is not easily accessible. Despite difficulties, language-brokering events are predictable in some sites more than others. For example, doctor–patient interactions are organized by schedules, allowing time to plan ahead.

I began with a general interest in the language brokering practice, not specifically concerned with the medical site. Drawing on my training in the ethnography of communication and my previous research and personal experiences, I designed the study as an ethnography of language brokering in the Arab American community. As I engaged more in my community of research, I decided to focus on a single interactional site, the multiparty interactions of medical visits. As such, this study is a hybrid between ethnography and sociological interpretive research; it began with the former and continued with the latter.

Medical sociology is traditionally concerned with examining the ways in which power structures are manifested in the doctor-patient relationship, influenced by the work of pioneer theoreticians, such as Talcott Parsons (1902–1979), Erving Goffman (1922–1982), and Anthony Giddens (1938–). This has been practiced mostly by building initial connections with medical sites to examine how healthcare providers carry out their professional duties. To illustrate this point, here are some excerpts of abstracts from the groundbreaking edited volume of John Heritage and Douglas W. Maynard, *Communication in Medical Care: Interaction between Primary Care Physicians and Patients* (2006): "This chapter . . . demonstrates that even subtle differences in how physicians design questions can change the action that questions perform" (Robinson, p. 23), "In this chapter, I examine the organization of closing in primary care visits" (West, p. 380), and "physicians exhibit not only that they are knowledgeable but *how* they are knowledgeable" (Maynard & Frankel, p. 252). Conducts of other interactional participants are certainly included when analyzing medical communications. For example, Tanya Stivers' chapter demonstrates that, "[I]n acute medical encounters, the final treatment decision is negotiated by physicians and parents" (p. 279). Nonetheless, medical sociological studies examine the healthcare system with an analytical lens focally directed at medical providers, which surely may include the responses they receive.

Ethnographic studies offer a rather panoramic lens. Even when the focus is on a single interactional site, researchers usually involve multiple community members and combine different research methodological tools that may or may not include field observation, recordings, and interviews. Even when the focus is on a single interactional site, researchers usually combine different methodologies, including some form of field observation, recording, and interviewing, and they involve different community members. Certainly, there is no single definition of ethnographical research, but it often involves a rather hybrid methodological paradigm, more than what is accustomed in CA interactional research. Ethnographies of immigrant communication, for example, are designed by building conducts with immigrant families and following them to different interactional sites, which may include medical settings and others. The works of Marjorie F. Orellana (2009, 2015), Inmaculada García Sanchez (2010, 2014), and Vikki Katz (2014 a & b) are excellent examples. In a study on language brokering among Latino families in Los Angeles, Katz interviewed physicians, child language brokers, and parents. Orellana and García Sanchez recorded real-life language-brokering activities at home and school conferences and observed immigrant families using their bilingual skills to build meaning-making in various everyday activities.

For this study, I began my research by visiting mosques, schools, and refugee organizations to spread word of mouth about my research. After securing a few participating families, I interviewed parents, children, and informally talked to a school principal, NGO director, psychologist, and doctor. I also observed without recordings in-home translation events of TV shows, mail, and medical and food labels. After a period of field observation and community engagement, my interests shifted to focus primarily on analyzing the forms of talk and the process of meaning-making in doctor–patient interactions, where language brokering demanded considerable coordinating efforts among family members, more than what appeared to be required for other regular daily translation events around the community. People also acted more naturally and intuitively in the healthcare context. The decision to focus on the practice of brokering medical interactions came organically in harmony with the community's specific characteristics.

Notably, however, the accessibility of recording due to the organization of the medical domain does not reflect the difficulties experienced by families, as they navigate the U.S. healthcare system and culture. Fortunately, the amiable relationships I built at the inception of data collection were quite productive in fashioning a smooth experience. While recording, families were comfortably engaging in their medical interactions without much ado about my camera or my presence.

On these accounts, studying brokered medical interactions as the primary site of my research was inspired by a few perspectives related to field development and my initial ethnographical efforts. These perspectives could be summarized as follows:

1. The limited work on the subject in related disciplines.
2. The intensity and serious consequences of brokering medical interactions.
3. My field observation in which medical visits emerged as the most urgent language-brokering zone.
4. The ordinariness by which people managed their medical-brokering interactions.

Other language-brokering contexts, such as translating at home and shopping malls, seemed to put the families in a compromising position, trying to control the exposure of familial details, or forging translation events so that I may obtain data. As generous and touching as that can be, I felt these incidents were a bit unnaturalistic and emotionally demanding. As an experiment, I left my recording equipment with one family to capture in-home translation events as they occur naturally, and I trained a family member on how to use them. The designated helper reported some difficulties that interfered with recording authentic translation, such as having the equipment ready at the onset of the translation event. Sometimes, he forgot the camera running, capturing family actions unrelated to translation, which angered his mother. These experimental recordings were not analyzed. Additionally, most participants were eager to solicit my help with medical-related information and presented medical visits as the main setting where translation is profoundly needed. These families live in communities where many services are provided by Arabic-speaking businesses, while medical providers are usually assigned by insurance companies. I hope these notes can aid future language-brokering ethnographers to find appropriate solutions.

In a six-month period, I collected data from medical encounters in specialists' clinics, primary care visits, and hospital emergency care. I then employed the CA method to make the cooperative and micro-procedural nature of building meaning-making analytically visible. The goal is to problematize common concepts of competency and participation upon which the medical staff fashions communications with immigrant patients.

Before recording medical interactions, I worked on building relationships with the families. We talked on the phone, gathered around food and tea times, exchanged memories about our home country, and discussed developing political and social scenes in Iraq. As they grew more comfortable in my presence, we began discussing arrangements for the data-collection trips. The families selected the doctors' visits I may attend, and I shared reliable contact information in case of last-minute changes. All participating families were kindly and gracefully welcoming. In one incident, I met the parents at their home and then drove together to collect their daughter, the family-designated language broker, from her high school, and then continued to their doctor's appointment. It felt rather similar to what I have done for my family. For those warm and genuine moments of sharing lives, I am forever grateful.

Then, my study began with a broad field involvement, but continued with a focal interest with a singular site, the mediated medical interaction. Nonetheless, throughout the chapters, the reader will meet the same families and know parts of their immigration trajectories, life stories, and medical histories. Some of their interactions are analyzed multiple times to serve different analytical objectives. In that vein, although this work was designed as an ethnography project, it was developed into a study with data collections and analyses rooted in the CA methodology. It analyzes social interactions in different medical settings and phases, while it continues to shed an ethnographic character on discussions by featuring medical cases and life narratives of the same limited number of families.

Observing and analyzing these quotidian experiences reveal many contextual challenges that ought to be part of the general medical experience of the immigrant population. For example, the language barrier may contribute to violating a long-standing field ethic, even if intentionally. We discussed previously a case in which the language broker was frustrated at seeing her mother, a former school principal in her home country, being moved around the examination room without being informed. We can easily recognize that the practice of informing patients before being subjected to a medical procedure, such as lifting sleeves to measure blood pressure or changing seats to sit closer to their medical examiner, is a standard practice in Western medicine.

Negotiating language and cultural difficulties and defying institutional norms so that to gain the right to interactional floors and access to healthcare benefits are primary challenges shared by most immigrant patients and their families. Some of the obstacles immigrant communications face challenge the boundaries of what we would let drift as acceptable and humane behavior.

A world of knowledge still needs to be unearthed regarding the impact of language disparities on immigrant medical interactions and medical outcomes; this book plants a seed in that direction.

THE COMMUNITY OF RESEARCH

Collecting language-brokering data began originally as a dissertation project that lasted about six months. In the summer of 2013, I began my fieldwork as a graduate researcher after receiving grants from the UCLA Graduate Mentorship Program and the UCLA Culture Brain and Development Program for a project on language brokering among Arabic-speaking communities in Southern California. I collected data from three sites: Los Angeles County, Orange County, and San Diego County. My original objective was to explore language-brokering characteristics in the Arab American community, focusing specifically on the impact of sociopolitical contexts on the language-brokering practice in public and private spheres. As explained above, after a few interviews and field trips, I found myself keenly interested in brokered medical interactions.

Iraqi immigrants arrived in the United States, and California specifically, in noticeable numbers in the mid-1970s and began establishing scattered communities around the Greater Los Angeles and San Diego counties. The larger flex of Iraqis began to arrive in the early 1990s propelled by the dangerous security and economic conditions in the aftermath of the many wars in Iraq's recent history, namely the Iraq-Iran war from 1980 to 1988, the Gulf war in 1990, the coalition war in 2003, and the sectarian violence in 2006.

A small set of data came from Orange County. A large Arab American community has built a local district called *Little Arabia* in Anaheim (figure 2.1), which has aided in making the county home to Arabs from all backgrounds, including a small population of Iraqi families residing mostly around Irvine and Anaheim (Nash, 2021). I accompanied a recent immigrant family, a mother and her daughter, from Irvine to a few shopping trips, and another family from Anaheim to medical visits; only the sample of data from the second family is included in this book.

Yet most of the ethnographic fieldwork and collected data came from the Iraqi community in El Cajon, San Diego, to which we will turn our attention.

El Cajon: Little Baghdad

El Cajon is a small urban city located 17 miles east of downtown San Diego, where diverse ethnic populations live over an area of 14.50 square miles, with 105,432 population. The city's population consists of 69.3 percent Whites, 27.1 percent Hispanics, 7.0 percent Black or

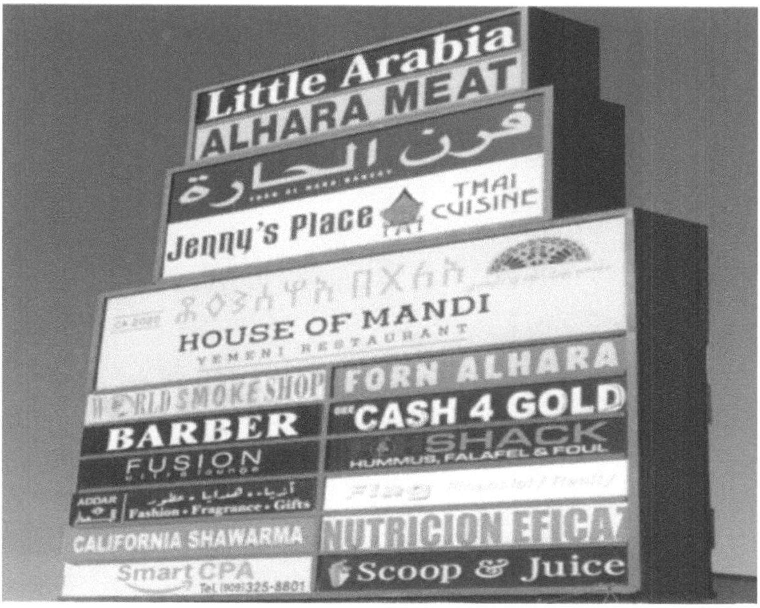

Figure 2.1 Little Arabia in Anaheim, Orange County. *Source:* Author.

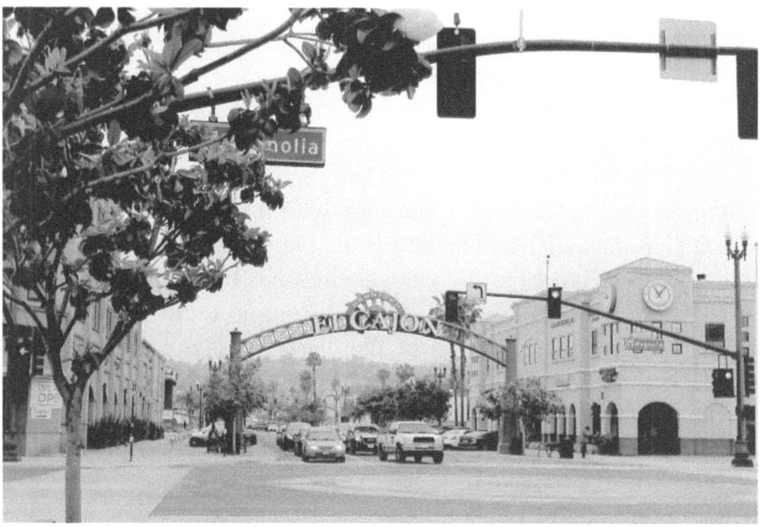

Figure 2.2 El Cajon City Where Little Baghdad Is Located around a Few Intersections between Magnolia and Main Streets. *Source:* Author.

African Americans, 4.5 percent Asians, plus other minority groups. The claimed percentage of Whites undoubtedly includes Middle Eastern people who are often listed in census surveys under the bubble, "White."

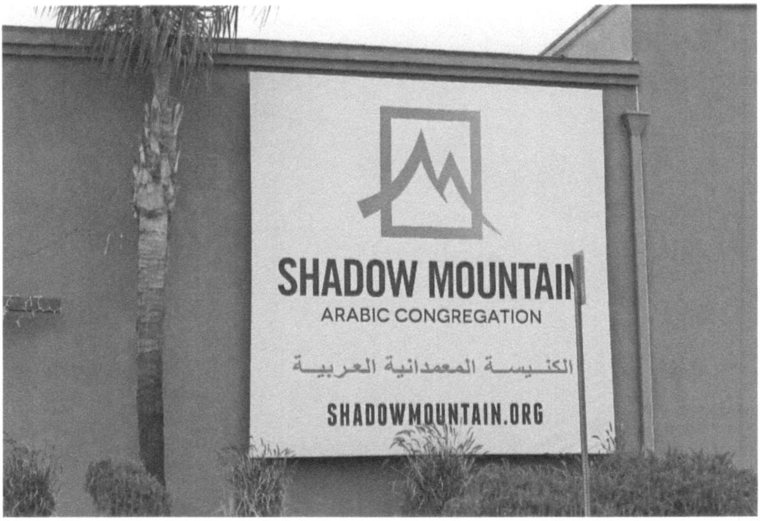

Figure 2.3 The Arabic Script Decorates Many of the City's Buildings and Streets, Such as This Church. *Source*: Author.

Twenty-eight percent of the city residents are foreign-born, with around 42.6 percent of five-year-olds and older speaking languages other than English at home. There are 9.4 percent of people with disabilities and 8 percent without health insurance.

The Iraqi community in El Cajon is home to the largest U.S.'s Chaldean Community after Detroit along with other diverse Iraqi ethnic and religious groups. The Chaldean community, a Catholic Christian group also referred to as ethnic Assyrians, makes up around 40,000 families of the city's total population (Holmes, 2020). The city is also home to considerable numbers of Mandaeans, a religious group whose religion is based on John the Baptist teaching; Kurds, an ethnic group from the Iraqi northern Kurdistan region; Turkmans, speakers of a version of the Turkish language originally from the oil-rich city of Kirkuk; and Muslims, mostly Shia, who also constitute another larger Iraqi group in El Cajon and other surrounding cities. The community centers mostly around an area known as Little Baghdad, located around intersections between the Main Street and Magnolia Street (figure 2.2), where the Arabic language and culture are visibly decorating the city landscape (figure 2.3). Little Baghdad is a busy district, richly populated with Iraqi restaurants, coffee and sweet shops, grocery stores, doctor offices, home-service businesses, beauty salons, jewelry shops, mosques, churches, Iraqi-owned gas stations, and even a small publishing company (figure 2.4a & b, figure 2.5a & b).

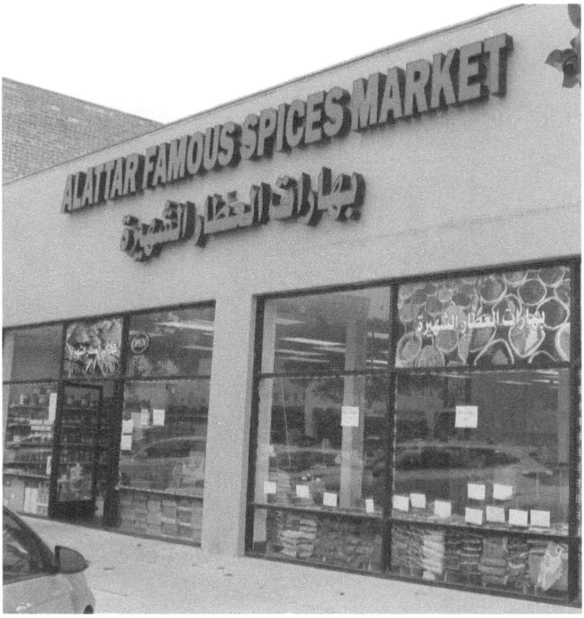

Figure 2.4A Middle Eastern Spices Shop. *Source:* Author.

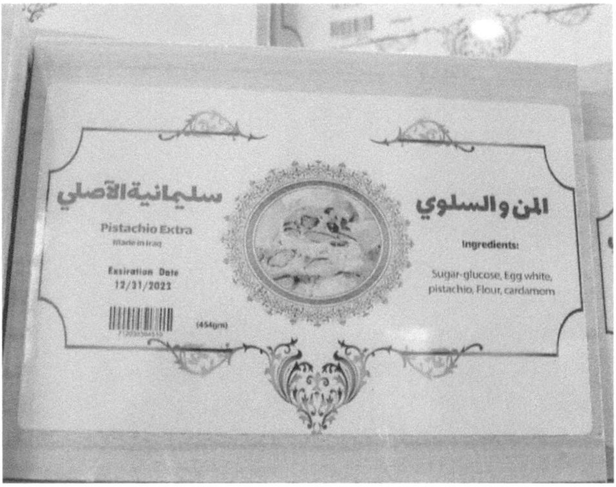

Figure 2.4B Sweets from Iraq in Royal Sweets Bakery and Coffee Shop, El Cajon. *Source:* Author.

I visited the Chaldean-Middle Eastern Social Service (CMSS) office in El Cajon, a nonprofit organization that provides a range of medical and immigrational services to local underserved communities. I interviewed the center's director and psychiatrist and witnessed the employees performing varied

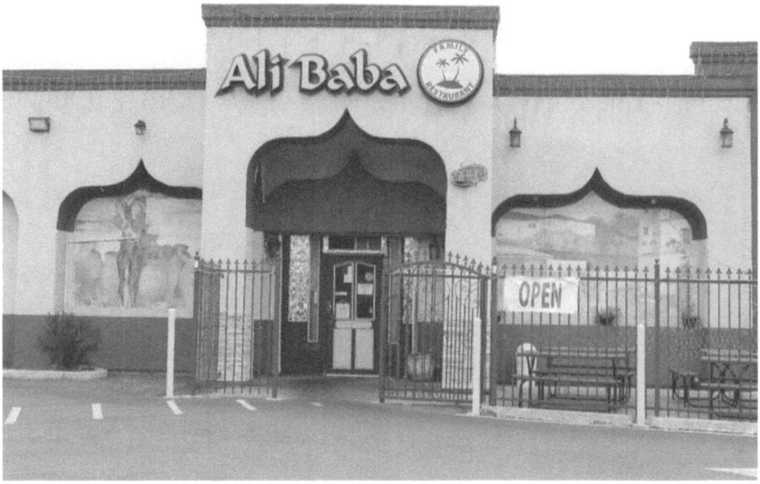

Figure 2.5A Ali Baba, a Popular Iraqi Restaurant in El Cajon. *Source:* Author.

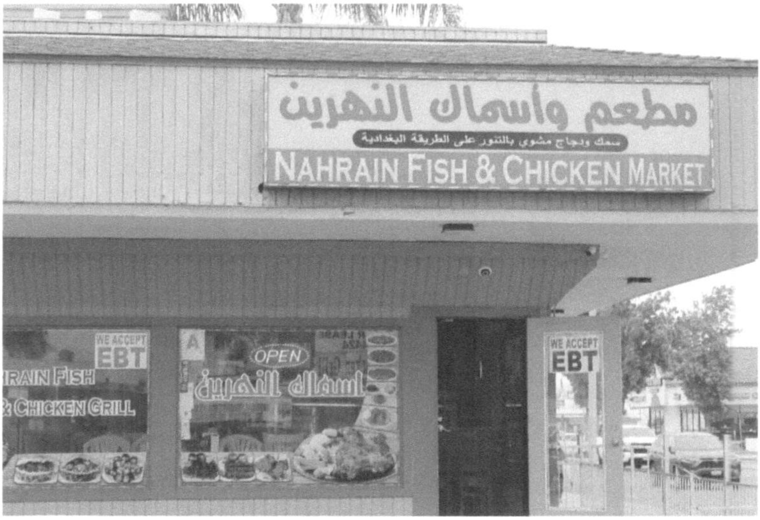

Figure 2.5B Al-Nahrain, a Popular Iraqi Restaurant in El Cajon. *Source:* Author.

services, such as assisting with job applications, immigration forms, and medical and insurance papers. During one of my visits, I observed a staff member helping a man with his job applications. His limited-English skills unlimited his agency. While providing information in his Christian Baghdadi dialect, he carefully observed the process of filling his job application and asked questions every time a slot was left empty. Witnessing his keen monitoring of the activity juxtaposed with frequently expressing gratitude toward the staff member was indeed humbling. His sharp gaze embodied a request to be included in all parts of the activity, which, in its essence, was a hope for security a decent living.

Participating Families

In that manner of field observations and community involvement, I met participating families. The analyses in this book draw on audio and video recordings from three families, two from San Diego and one from Orange County. All participants received pseudonyms and consent forms. The teenage language brokers received consent forms in English that were explained and signed in their parents' presence. Parents (the patients) and the adult language brokers signed consent forms prepared in Arabic.

Family 1 (Amal and Nada)

I met Nada in the hallway of CMSS where she sat next to a middle-aged lady, her aunt—as I learned later. While waiting, Nada also helped other people in queues. Her inclination to help others encouraged me to approach the couple and introduce myself. In Arabic, Nada immediately explained that she translates frequently for her parents, siblings, relatives, and even neighbors. I asked to speak to her parents requesting their permission to participate in my study. As such, we exchanged contact information before parting. Later that day, I received a phone call from Nada's mother, Amal, who gave her consent of participation. I met the family a few times at their home in El Cajon, before scheduling data-collection trips, where I met both parents, their four children, and the grandfather who lived with the family. In one of my visits, I was lucky to witness how the family orchestrated the meaning-making of a phone call about furniture delivery, beautifully accomplished by the two teenage sisters and parents.

The mother, Amal, is a 36-year-old Christian from Mosul, a city in the north of Iraq. After marriage, she lived in Baghdad where all of her four children were born. The family left Iraq to Turkey where they lived three years before immigrating to the United States. The family's youngest child, a four-year-old girl, was born in Iraq, just before fleeing the country due to the violence and social unrest following the 2003 war. At the time of meeting the family, the child had a condition of speech delay that resulted, as the mother believed, from the trauma of moving and relocating multiple times before settling in SD.

Amal married her high-school sweetheart right after their graduation, and both received no further education. In Baghdad, the family lived in a neighborhood close to other relatives. Missing cousins and family gatherings was the biggest drawback of immigration for the children, as they contended. Whereas managing work and life in an unfamiliar culture without family support was the daily challenge their parents had to navigate. Upon arriving in San Diego, Amal attended adult English classes inconsistently, because the classes were crowded and unsuccessfully taught, as she explained. Instead, she found a part-time job in a local Iraqi bakery to help with the family expenses while her husband worked full-time in hotel maintenance. The two older children also had part-time jobs while attending school and helping with familial responsibilities. Amal's oldest child, Nada, is the designated language broker.

Nada is a seventeen-year-old high-school student who has three siblings, a sixteen-year-old sister, a fourteen-year-old brother, and a four-year-old sister. The three older children speak Arabic, Chaldean, and English, while the youngest child understands and speaks a few words of Chaldean, the language of interaction at home. The older siblings have developed functional proficiencies in English allowing them to manage their schoolwork and job duties independently. Despite their English skills, the mother depends on Nada to translate the medical visits of all family members.

Nada finds brokering as a natural form of family help necessary to survive in their new home country. Except when interfering with school duties, mediating family needs at home and elsewhere unburdened Nada. The support she receives from her high-school teachers and staff is crucial in managing her school, job, and home responsibilities successfully. Her teachers, as she explained, never denied her the opportunity of making up late assignments and meeting after regular school hours to catch up on missed work. Nada also helps neighbors and relatives voluntarily and has convinced her father to rely on her instead of friends or professional services as he was more inclined to do. Her work as a community language broker has inspired Nada to pursue a career in medicine. At the time of the study, Nada was enrolled in an after-school program through her high school that prepares her for a future career in nursing.

Family 2 (Salma and Hamid)

The second family in this study also lived in El Cajon, another Christian family originally from Mosul but lived in Baghdad before immigrating to the United States. The family consists of a middle-aged couple whose two adult children, at the time of the interview, were in the process of relocating from back home, and the wife's mother, Salma. Salma is a seventy-seven-year-old woman who came from Baghdad a few months before our meeting. Salma and her son, Hamid, became my second participating family.

In Baghdad, Salma cared for and lived with her two adult grandchildren whose mother, Salma's daughter, passed away. That separation hurt Salma the most. Her eyes filled with tears and travelled frequently to meet their photos placed on the nearby end table. Salma appeared in good health and energy except for moderately age-related issues controlled by medicine, such as blood pressure, high cholesterol, and hearing loss. I recorded five visits with the hearing-aid clinician and two visits with an eye doctor. Salma's medical visits are translated by her son, Hamid.

Hamid is in his early fifties, married with one college-student daughter, and lived with his family at the same apartment complex where his sister and mother lived. He arrived in San Diego five years before I met the family after receiving asylum status for serving as a translator during the 2003 war on Iraq. Many people who helped the coalition forces with translation or other informative roles received death threats from local oppositional groups, which promoted the United States and other European countries to relocate members of this group outside of Iraq. Hamid's English skills were still developing at the time of our meetings, generally lacking some grammar points and specialized vocabulary, which in turn affected how he translated his mother's medical visits. In response to a question about life in the diaspora, Hamid conveyed that he was content to secure good living and security conditions for his family but missed his house, friends, and work.

Family 3 (Karim and Nathen)

The third family in this study was a personal relative. Karim was a seventy-three-year-old Muslim from Baghdad who lived in Orange County with his son, Nathen, and his family. Karim was generally healthy and led an active physical and mental lifestyle with daily walks and keen observation of world-developing news. He had mild age-related conditions of diabetes and high blood pressure managed by medicine and diet. I recorded a few in-home translation events of reading mail, medicine labels, phone calls, TV programs, and immigration letters by different members of his family. I also recorded doctor visits and observed phone calls with pharmacists. Contrary to other study participants, Karim did not necessarily have a designated language broker. Instead, he solicited the help of his adult children, whoever was available.

Nathan is a forty-five-year-old father of three young children at the time of data collection. His father's primary doctor is an Arabic-speaking provider which limits the need for regular translation. Nevertheless, Nathen, and his siblings, took Karim to his medical appointments and translated interactions with pharmacists, nurses, and occasional conduct with English-speaking providers. Nathen was confident in his English abilities, and that influenced the manner in which he managed his father's medical needs.

LANGUAGE AND TRANSCRIPTIONS

The Iraqi dialect covers many varieties, spoken by about 40 million people in a geographical area of about 438,052 square kilometers. Iraqis are mostly Muslims but also followers of other religions such as Christians, Mandeans, Yazidis, Shabak, and others. The Iraqi dialect, also known as the Mesopotamian dialect, is generally divided into two varieties: Gilit Arabic and Geltu Arabic—the names are derived from their equivalent formal Arabic phrase "I said." The Gilit dialects is a cluster of varieties spoken along the Tigris to which the speech norms of Baghdad and other surrounding areas belong. The Geltu dialect is the Euphrates cluster of spoken varieties used in the northern part of the country and along the Euphrates. The spoken varieties of Mosul are versions of the Geltu; thus, this dialect is often referred to as the Maslawi Arabic. Historically, these two varieties are also associated with religion: the Gilit variety represents Muslims and the Geltu variety represents Christians and Jews (Blanc, 1964).

There are more sounds in the Iraqi dialect than in the formal Arabic, and English. Besides the shared twenty-eight consonants with the formal Arabic, there are additional consonants in the Iraqi dialect, گ /g/ and چ /ğ/. The گ /g/ sound replaces its equivalent in the formal Arabic /q/—although not comprehensively; while چ / ĵ/ is used as a variation of ج / j/, and ڤ/v/ appears in borrowing words, such as the female name, ڤيان. Iraqi Arabic has more vowels than the formal Arabic, with five long vowels (ā, ē, y, ō, and ū), three short vowels (a, i, and u), and two semi-vowels (w and y) (Erwin, 2004). Appendix 1 contains two tables: table A1 describes the Iraqi consonants, and table A2 describes the vowels.

Transcription

The speakers in this study represent both the Gilit and the Geltu varieties of the Iraqi dialect. One family is a Muslim family from Baghdad, while the other two are Christians from Mosul, but all the families came from Baghdad and are familiar with the standard Baghdadi dialect. Hamid and his mother mixed between the Geltu and Gilit varieties, reflecting their mixed backgrounds as originally from the north but lived in the capital.

I organized the transcripts in three-line turns as numbered in the manner demonstrated below:

01: اللغة العربية—an Arabic script turn
1a: fii alluga al'rabiya—an Arabic transliteration turn
1b: A translation turn

The transliteration depicts the way the speakers used their Arabic and English skills; therefore, it contains original errors, mixed and awkward utterances. Through my translation, I tried to preserve some of the unusual Arabic syntax as used by the participants; I believe these incidents reflect the intense emotional and linguistic demands of mediating and interacting in crosslinguistic medical contexts. To preserve the details of face-to-face interactions as they occur in real-time interactions, I used the transcribing system of CA (Hepburn & Bolden, 2012), which was originally developed by Gail Jefferson and described by Sacks, Schegloff, and Jefferson (1974), but I also created a few conventions to match the script of the Arabic language. For example, I stretch the shape of the letter to represent lengthening sounds and I do that by pressing the letter and shift keys simultaneously on the Arabic keyboard. Appendix 2 explains the CA symbols and other conventions used in this study.

DATA ANALYSIS

The theoretical foundations and empirical approaches of CA are the methods I adopted to study the collected videos and audios of brokering Iraqi English medical interactions (Sacks, Schegloff, & Jefferson, 1974). CA examines social interactions in all contexts of social life as "primordial means through which the business of the social world is transcribed, the identities of its participants are affirmed or denied and its cultures as transmitted, renewed, and modified" (Goodwin & Heritage, 1990, p. 283). Influenced by the pioneer work of Erving Goffman (1922–1982) and John J. Gumperz (1922–2013), sociologists, anthropologists, linguists, and cognitive psychologists concur in studying face-to-face interaction as a strategic site for examining human action and cognition. We perform situational roles and competencies only by giving close attention to the local organization of how talk is initiated, organized, developed, and closed. As a generic approach to studying these interactional mechanisms in everyday conversations, CA operational tools are oriented by four assumptions:

1. All types of casual and institutional interactions are structurally organized.
2. Interlocutors' contributions are doubly contextualized; they are both context-shaped and context-renewed.
3. No interactional details are dismissed readily as disorderly or irrelevant.
4. Studying social interaction is approached through data collected from audio and video recordings of real-life conversations.

Through these fundamental elements, CA analyses show how all interactions are sequentially organized and how their constitutive actions display contextual relevancies in the way of building understanding cooperatively (Goodwin, 2018). For example, Harvey Sacks ushered in the seminal work of CA as a rigorous and systematic method for analyzing the micro-procedural laborious actions by showing how callers and listeners orient their attention around the regularity of concealing or providing personal identities when reaching out to suicide-prevention hotline.

People enter a conversation with a broad array of personal traits, circumstances, and backgrounds; whether these elements are known or unknown to conversation partners is beyond the point of how CA unfolds human actions and intentions. We cannot really speak of people's intentions, simply because intentions are invisible entities; we can, however, note the ways in which intentions are carried out in the form of speech. The method is mostly concerned with how a turn of talking is designed and how actions are treated as relevant to its context. Through this methodological approach, human cognition is pragmatically displayed by making the enactment of understanding and misunderstanding and the structure of alignment and misalignment analytically visible. The absence of an action is equally expressive and observable. For example, a couple may have the following conversation:

1	A:	Are you going to work?
2	B:	Yes.
3	A:	Ok.

In this hypothetical situation, A asks a question geared toward a future event, B offers a minimal response to A's question that is relevant to the purpose of A's inquiry. A's intent is vague and may raise a host of possibilities about the circumstances for A's question, but B chooses to respond concisely. A longer episode may reveal A's intention of asking or B's reason for giving a cursory response, but the above sequence is sufficient to display the projectivity of future actions as available to interlocutors, analysts, and readers. Natural conversations are messy and may extend to multiple turns, but the above sequence is intended to show, in the simplest form, the meaning of studying the relevancy between turns of talking. Upon receiving the desired information, A closes the conversation with a minimum item, *Okay*. The verbal and nonverbal components (the latter is not considered in the example here) of A's utterances and the ways in which B displays an orientation toward such details are the concerns of CA researchers. The objective is to show how actions in the ordinary and departed forms are accomplished. If both dimensions are analytically visible, then "the empirical task of showing that a particular normative organization is operative in interaction will have been achieved" (Heritage, 1988, p. 131).

Actions, as in the example above, are analyzed through the concept of *adjacency pairs* (Sacks, Schegloff, & Jefferson, 1974), which central assumption demonstrates the relatedness between its first part—FPP (e.g., the first part of a greeting or invitation), and its second part—SPP (e.g., a response to a greeting or invitation). Heritage (1988) notes that the relationship between the two parts shows how "each turn is addressed to the matters raised by the turn preceding" (p. 129). Daily interactions are parts, they may include a pre-sequence to set the stage for the base action, insert-sequence turns to ask or add information, and a post-sequence turns to close, extend, or start a new topic.

CA is a research stream born out of ethnomethodology with a primary concern to studying the commonsense reasoning skills and abilities through which the ordinary members of a culture produce and recognize intelligible courses of actions (Heritage, 1984). It pragmatically unpacks the philosophy of John L. Austin (1975) on how language, as a means of carrying human thoughts, feelings, and intentions, perform actions. In other words, CA is concerned with the systematic ways in which forms of questions, offerings, disagreements, invitations, and other actions are designed to achieve their objectives and how these actions are received and reciprocated.

The power of this method in making human competencies, actions, and intentions visible resides in the use of real-life data, giving the reader the opportunity to see how the interaction is unfolded as closely as when it actually happened. This is certainly profoundly different from reporting and experimental research. The CA method proposes to inform understandings on the production and recognition of intelligible course of actions, while reporting reflects experiences from recollections, and experimental research produces knowledge in controlled environments.

A key element in CA is the attention to micro-features of talk-in-interactions, such as overlaps, repairs, volume, pitch, and gaze. These fine-grained interactional details show the subtlety of transferring knowledge that participants treat as relevant. Through these micro-procedural actions, interlocutors pull on an array of background and situational information to build relatedness. The mechanism of receiving and delivering such actions is most effective when it is designed in consideration of the recipient's episteme, a concept referred to as "recipient design"; it is the ability to tailor a communicative behavior to a particular addressee (Garfinkel, 1964). A break of communication occurs when the recipient's knowledge is not taken into consideration in the design of utterances. For example, if a doctor fails to consider his patient's knowledge or understanding by using unfamiliar medical terms without explanation, the patient might produce verbal or nonverbal actions that make the doctor's unaccountability to the process of building mutual meaning-making, a situation that may contribute to patients' satisfaction negatively.

The language barrier combined with cultural asymmetries and unbalanced authoritative roles in institutional settings, the concern of this book, create critical obstacles in the process of building mutual intelligibility. To discern how these features operate in shaping participatory patterns in brokered medical encounters, we consider the following questions: Do medical providers structure their talk in ways that account for the patients' understanding, or would they deliver their message by relying heavily on the language broker with whom they share a level of linguistic commonality? With these research questions in mind, I aim to impart knowledge on how limited-English-speaking patients respond to doctors' talk when their talk is delivered via the language broker; how they manage to embed themselves in the interaction when they do not receive translation, and how they manage to exercise their patienthood within the discursive asymmetrical layers of institutional and brokering discourses.

CONCLUSION

I dedicate this final section to sharing with my readers, especially the researcher among them, a few thoughts about the methodological way of studying human behavior. Duranti (2004) notes that the artificial separation among the fields of social sciences has limited its progress and influence. A social scientist's field of study is the development of human thought and its pragmatic enactment. How this scientific burden is carried out is a thing of methodology, which unfairly, to researchers and examined cultures, should be dogmatically determined beforehand.

I went into the field as an ethnographer, but my field of research demanded a specific ethnomethodological context of study. The start and development of my research were organically shaped. I began my language-brokering journey with studies designed by open-ended interview and survey methods. I investigated the impact of widespread ideologies associated with Arab and Muslim communities in zones of contact where different world views, personal investments, linguistic and cultural abilities, and generational values interact. To get deeper into the topic, I designed a study that took me inside people's homes and allowed me to share trips to schools, mosques, shopping malls, and medical visits. The needs of the research community, however, led my study to examine patterns of participation that are relevant to the general immigrant-patient populations.

Ethnography has emerged in the late nineteenth century and was developed by British, French, and American anthropologists as a tool to study human cultures and social structures. Although it is acknowledged as Western tradition, its ways of collecting data have long been practiced among non-Western cultures. A critical difference between the two spheres lies in the perspectives through which knowledge is produced. The Western thinker set out to look for *the truth*, influenced by the domination of the Church on the formation of the Western thoughts and society, while non-Western scholars went out to understand norms of living and expressions of life. The scope of the former forces understandings from that limited lens, whereas the latter is descriptive and naturalistic in its essence. As the practice developed into a systematic discipline, it became the primary method of gathering information on non-Western practices and communities.

The methodological approaches of CA that were developed into a systematic discipline in the 1970s and have since been practiced in the United States, Europe, and increasingly in other parts of the world somewhat frees beforehand unacknowledged prejudices by focusing on locally and sequentially managed actions. Social structures are sustained insofar as their constitutive elements are manifested practically through daily interactions. The elements of these interactions become doubly contextual; they shape and are shaped by linguistic and social contexts. Thus, interactions bear the potentiality, as well as the responsibility, of shaping the present and changing the future. Paying attention to this revoicing and dialogical nature of interactions allows observants to witness how actions are recognized through subtle, cooperative, and orderly micro-procedures. Harold Garfinkel argues, "[W]hat makes an action recognizable to others as an action of a particular sort of constitutive aspect of the orderliness of action—a sequential and reflective order" (Garfinkel, 2008, p. 19). The CA method is concerned with studying the phenomenon of orderly actions, regardless of the setting or the number of occurrences, to establish the development of understanding, identity performance, and situational competency. Witnessing the process of building understandings in same-language interactions is a sublime opportunity to study the orderly formation of actions. Observing how these processes conjure in crosslinguistic interactions where people negotiate diverse layers of historical, cultural, and linguistic norms is indeed marvelous.

Scholars go into the field equipped with the knowledge, methodologies, and research questions backed by years of training and education. Yet the privilege of observing the capacity of micro-actions in influencing the trajectory of conversation obligates an open-minded and a humble readiness to adjust primary plans to the demands of the research ground. In that manner, the methodological ways of producing understandings allow the context of change to be born.

Chapter 3

Patients' Initiatives

Building Patienthood Cooperatively and Independently

This chapter deals with actions in which the Iraqi patients in this study manage their medical visits by initiating actions that challenge the discursive forms of linguistic, cultural, and situational asymmetries. Two types of initiating actions are distinguished: (1) conventional actions formed by working with the brokering practice, performed in Arabic, and (2) deviant actions enacted by overriding the brokering process to respond directly to doctors' questions, often in English. Both types of actions, conventional and deviant initiatives, redirect the LB turn-taking system and alter participatory patterns.

Scholars note that structured social interactions yield anomalous patterns, recognized as a deviant-case analysis, operating outside the parameters of what is considered a conventional order of talking (Sacks, Schegloff, & Jefferson, 1974; Schegloff, 1968). Though they challenge the boundaries of acceptability and normalcy, these actions are common affairs even when social norms are institutionally regulated. This chapter locates two methods of patients' initiative actions: conventional actions formed in the first pair part (FPP) and unconventional actions formed in the second pair part (SPP). Some initiations are found to be constituted by transgressing the language assistance turn to activate fluid contextual roles. Both types of initiated actions, however, alter participatory roles and redirect the LB turn-taking system. The argument for the type of initiated actions identified in this chapter is specific to the LB context as a site marked with linguistic, cultural, and social challenges. Identifying limited-English-speaking patients' actions as initiatives is irrelevant to their sequential location, as they may come in first, second, or extended positions. Their construction with or without translation by employing different semiotic resources, manipulating language abilities, and altering the turn-taking sequence is the locus of studying patients' initiatives in this chapter.

The doctor–patient interaction is traditionally conceptualized as a formal interview in which the doctor is the interviewer posting questions, and the patient is the interviewee providing answers, a pattern that claimed to steer the interactional progressivity toward institutionally determined structures and goals (Cohen-Cole, 1991; Mishler, 1984). These constraints that influence same-language encounters are equally operational in crosslinguistic encounters. In that vein, brokered doctor–patient interactions exhibit the potential to be constrained by two types of discursive structures: the institutional discourse—enacted by the physician—and the brokering discourse—enacted by the family broker. But, do limited-English-speaking patients passively comply with these constraints? If they deviate, what interactional resources aid their deviations? Also, how these actions are received? This chapter navigates these questions around the analyses of limited-English-speaking patients' initiatives to examine the fluid actuation of contextual identities and competencies in asymmetrical interactional contexts.

ACTION INITIATION

Initiating actions are commonly addressed by the interactional structure of adjacency pair, in which a relation between its parts constitutes "the most powerful device for relating utterances" (Sacks, 1992, p. 554). The concept of adjacency pair is quite simple, but its paucity resides in its pragmatic display of understanding and attention. People initiate actions to solicit human contact, achieve personal investments, and carry out the human instinct of socialization. Within the two parts, the FPP, where a speaker initiates an action, and the SPP, where another speaker responds, the SPP is investigated as a prismoid to the organization of relatedness in turns-in-interactions. Regarding FPPs, the design of turns is a common concern, such as the ways in which a sequence is initiated to enact a greeting (Sacks, 1992), self-correction versus being corrected by others (Drew, 1997), to express solidarity (Clayman, 2002), to offer a self-correction versus being corrected by others (Heritage & Sefi, 1992), or to preform self-praising as opposed to receiving a praise (Pomerantz, 1978).

In the medical context, actions are commonly initiated by doctors when collecting information to evaluate cases at hand; albeit patients may also initiate actions through questions and comments. Nevertheless, alternative patterns of action initiations are also noted. When discussing different types of initiatives, Jeffery Robinson (2001) argues that previous studies have conflated the impact of exogenous and endogenous variables in shaping patterns of asymmetries in institutional settings. Conversely, he suggests examining asymmetries in the light of the unique internal characteristics of an interaction as structured by participants' agency and language constraints. Frankel (1990) posits that forms of continuous talk can be examined as a locus for studying initiatives whether they are acknowledged with a response or ignored. These alternative views on action initiation have guided my understanding of limited-English-speaking patients' actions.

In this chapter, I analyze the ways in which Iraqi patients strike a balance between states of independency and co-participation in their ways of building patienthood around the discursive institutional and brokering structures. The default form of initiation in LB interactions are constructed in similar ways to the sequential order of initiatives in same-language interactions, with the patient occupying the first position of a sequence. Some of their occupancies are delivered through language-brokering assistance, while others override the brokering process to constitute speakership independently without translation or solicitation. These actions challenge the discursive cultural and linguistic asymmetries inherent in mediated medical encounters.

BROKERING DISCOURSE AND ACTION INITIATION

The default layout of brokering discourse is constituted by duplicated turns, a bilingual uptake after each monolingual turn. When conceptualizing the language-brokering sequence in terms of adjacency pairs, the structure below resembles the generic LB turn-taking system: (R for rendition, 1 for the dominant language, and 2 for the heritage language):

A: A doctor's turn, FPP-1
B: A language broker's rendition, FPP-R-2
C: A language brokeree's responsive turn, SPP-2
D: A language broker's rendition of SPP-2, SPP-R-1
E: A doctor's sequence-closing or sequence-expansion turn in 1.

The above pattern is considered the conventional LB turn-taking system, and the expected and normative manner by which the language mediation is performed, especially in institutional interactions. If actions are initiated by patients, rather than doctors, the above pattern is reversed. Cecila Wadensjö (2014), however, notes that mediated discourse is marked by non-normative, more than normative, patterns, with the former clearly displays the cooperative and interactive nature of the mediator's work.

In the collected Iraqi data, many patients' initiations are accomplished by the normative brokering structure in the form of FPP-2 → FPP-R-1 → SPP-1 → SPP-R-2. Some of these initiatives, however, stop at the levels of FPP2, when patients' initiations are left without response, or FPP2-SPP2, when patients' talk is answered by the language broker. In this pattern, patients ask questions, request information, and offer alternative accounts for their conditions. These conventional initiatives bear a threefold value: They activate their social membership categories as:

1. A language brokeree in their choice of depending on family interpreters.
2. A parent by designating a language broker among their bilingual relatives.
3. A patient based on their agency, not doctors' agency, which claimed to govern the progressivity of doctor–patient interactions.

This chapter exemplifies both types of initiated actions, albeit putting more analytical weight on deviant cases constituted by overriding the brokering process to activate a complicated set of contextually relevant interactional competencies.

Conventional Initiated Actions

The below fragment exemplifies a conventionally formed initiation, performed dyadically in the form of FPP-2 → SPP-2, a sequence of talk between the language brokeree and the language broker in their heritage language. The patient, Karim, initiates an action while the doctor gets ready to perform a small medical procedure on Karim's elbow:

Excerpt (1): Kar: Karim/patient, NAT: Nathen/son/language broker.

```
282   KAR: بَلكي تنجح هاي.
282a       balki tnjaḥ hāi.
282b       Hopefully this works.

283        (0.1)

284   NAT: تنجح،
284a       tnjaḥ,
284b       It works,

285   KAR: هو يگول ماكو مُشكلة بيها،
285a       hwa ygūl makū muškila byha,
285b       He says there is nothing wrong with it,

286   NAT: هو يگول وحدة ورى وحدة. يعني إذا مَصارت هاي تصير ذيج.
286a       hwa yg̱ūl waḥda wara waḥda. yʿni ʾiḏa maṣārt hāi tṣyr ḏyğ.
286b       He says one after the other. so if this didn't wcrk,
           that one does.
```

In line 282, Karim wishes that the scheduled procedure will treat his case successfully; a confirmation of his wish is given by his son (line 284). The act of confirmation, in its essence, is an emotional solidarity, solidifying the father's wish for a successful treatment built by the proper utility of the Arabic grammar. Nathen designs a culturally common manner of confirmation, formed by repeating the important item from the previous turn; in this case, it is the verbal form تنجح، /tnjaḥ/ [It works], which is an imperfective form that heightens the immediacy of actions (Brustad, 2000). Similarly, in line 286, Nathen presents the doctor's plan as a foreseeable course of action, using the perfect verb that denotes an aspect of a completed process, مَصارت /maṣārt/ [an attached negative marker *ma* + past tense verb *ṣārt*—did not work], and continues with a turn constructional unit (TCU) of an imperfect clause تصير ذيج /tṣyr ḏyǧ/ [present tense + demonstrative—that one works], adding an aspect of immediacy and assurance to an expected event in the near future, the event of a successful recovery. Karim's request for a confirmation of the doctor's evaluation as a benign case is designed by a simple interrogative (line 285). He receives an overall plan's summary, a sort of a quick recap suggesting that the proposed options are available and ordered based on the recovery process. In this case, Karim leads a dyadic exchange in Arabic by occupying the silence due to the doctor's engagement.

In a similar manner, Amal, the patient in the excerpt below, gives some possible medical reasons for her condition as her doctor engages with documenting his recommendation plan. This encounter is not scheduled to give new complaints. It is a meeting with a specialist to discuss results of an MRI exam upon which the doctor may design a treatment plan. Nonetheless, the patient finds it relevant to express some symptoms that she believes to be related to her condition. Her turn is designed by an imperative statement with a reporting-speech code 'gūli la' [tell him], in which she directs her daughter to transfer her hypotheses to the doctor:

Excerpt (2): AMA: Amal—the patient, NAD: Nada—the daughter/language broker

83 AMA: گولي له، يعني مو الُمشكلة من المفاصل مال زُگبة مالتي؟
83a gūli la, yʿni mū lmuškila min lmafāṣl mālrugba malti?
83b Tell him, so the problem is not from my neck joints?

84 تضرب على راسي.
84a tḍrub ʿla rāsi.
84b Pounding in my head.

85 (0.4)

86 NAD: °wait

87 AMA: أنـي-هـاي الاشهر عيوني تـغوش، تـغوش هوايـة.
87a āni-hāi aššhur ʿyūni tġawš, tġawš hwaya.
87b I-these months my eyes are blurry, very blurry.

88 (0.2)

89 AMA: هسّة شراح يسوي؟
89a hassa šrāḥ ysawi?
89b What is he going to do now?

In this fragment, the patient requests an engagement with her doctor by providing reasons that could be accountable for her condition—a case of severe headaches that promoted her primary care provider, in a previous visit, to order the MRI test and the meeting with the neurologist. The reported-speech code ‘gūli la’ [tell him] activates Amal’s language brokeree’s and parent’s roles by summoning her daughter to act in the capacity of brokering. Her turn receives a waiting request after a period of silence, constituting a no-translation action known as non-rendition (Wadensjö , 2014). The patient then alters her strategy and states that her eyes have been extremely blurry (line 88), a medical issue that should warrant transability. Amal requests a direct engagement with her doctor via the brokering sequence, but when her multiple attempts are denied, she submits to the gatekeeping position as enacted by her daughter in this segment by requesting the daughter’s understanding of the doctor’s plan.

In this example, Amal initiates requests of engagement by three methods: a direct request through an imperative, a tacit request through revealing a medical problem, and an indirect request through seeking the daughter’s understanding of the doctor’s plan. All these actions, however, fail to constitute a triadic sequence on the basis of the patient’s initiative. Unclear reasons could have contributed to deflating the patient’s efforts, such as experiencing language difficulty or observing the meeting’s progressivity that has reached a conclusion.

Amal continues to evaluate the ongoing interaction and builds more initiatives as she finds necessary. In the excerpt below, she initiates question–answer sequences to collect important information about her treatment plan:

Excerpt (3):

121 AMA: ها؟ <و>,مال عيون، شوكِت نروح عَليه؟
121a hā? <w>::mal ʿyūn, šwakit nrūḥ ʿalyh?
121b Ha? <and> the one for the eyes, when we’ll go to see him?

122 NAD: what about the eyes, like [the eye °specialist
123 DOC: [oh I’m gonna ask the girls to
124 set up an appointment=
125 NAD: =Awkay=

126 AMA: =وهاي-الدكتور-اه اه وين حَيكون؟ هذا الطبيب.=
126a =whāi-lductōr-ah ah- wēn ḥykūn? hāḏa lṭabyb.=

```
126b        =And this doctor-ah ah where is he going to be? this
            physician.=

127  NAD:   =يا طبيب؟
127a        =yā ṭabyb?
127b        =What physician?

128  AMA:   مال أبو العيون؟
128a        māl abū l‘yūn?
128b        The eye specialist?
```

In the above fragment, the patient attentively follows the visit's progress and intervenes to request missing information. She agentively gathers what has been received, what is still needed, and what deserves adding. In line 121, Amal asks about the time to visit the eye specialist, an earlier doctor's recommendation. Nada delivers the question, receives the answer, but does not relay the information back to her mother. Perhaps, Nada treats the doctor's answer as an action of her responsibility—knowing that she would be the person to arrange and mediate that visit, a sample of actions through which brokers explicitly and implicitly coordinate the ongoing interaction as well as future anticipated translating duties. Amal then asks about the location of the eye doctor. In line 127, the language broker asks, "What doctor?" revealing that Amal, not Nada, keeps up with the visits' details and progressivity.

The World Health Organization (WHO) recommends that patients should be educated prior to any type of procedure with all relevant operational details and time to recovery. The medical staff should also check on patients' fears and understanding. In the above examples, we saw our patient requesting relevant pieces of information that ought to be delivered as part of preparing her for upcoming steps. Similarly, the excerpt below takes place before administrating a procedure of treating an injured area and reveals that the patient himself requests essential pieces of information about his treatment procedure.

Excerpt (4):

```
269    DOC:    we take some fluid out.

270    NAT:    نسحب السائل هسّة.
270a           nsḥab assā'il hassa.
270b           We pull the fluid out now.

271            (0.1)
272    DOC:    okay?
273    NAT:    okay.

274    KAR:→   بنج يرادلها شي؟
274a           banj yrādlha ši?
```

274b Does it need an anesthetization or something?

275 NAT: are you gonna numb the area? Or,

276 DOC: we gonna put some coo:ling solutions,

277 NAT: راح نخلي فد شي مُبَرِد للمَنطقة،
277a rāḥ nxali fad ši mubarid ll-manṭaqa,
277b We're going to put some cooling thing on the area,

Our concern in this chapter is making patients' initiatives visible, those that have been overshadowed by inherent forms of discursive asymmetries. In line 269 above, the doctor informs that he plans to pull some fluid out of the injured area. The language broker translates the turn rather faithfully in line 270. The doctor then checks for understanding or agreement and receives confirmation from the language broker. In line 274, Karim, the patient, requests a vital piece of information, if the condition requires a numbing treatment to manage associated pain. Usually, this type of information is communicated as part of preparing the patient for a procedure. Neglecting to provide relevant details about the treatment promotes the patient to fish for them.

In the previous examples, we found our patients agentively initiating actions and leading the information-gathering process through the assistance of their language brokers. Sometimes, these actions are halted in their tracks toward triadic engagement when their turns are left untranslated or handled directly by the language brokers. The second section of the chapter identifies actions in which patients transgress the language-assistance turns to enact their patienthood independently.

Independently Initiated Actions

The phenomenon we unpack in this section is a deviant-case analysis in which limited-English-speaking patients diverge from dependency on the brokering process. Defining these actions as initiatives is unnecessarily restricted by the sequential order of the adjacency-pair structure. In other words, their constitution as initiatives is not linked to their sequential allocation as the first part of a sequence. They are a form of context-specific actions constructed by the ability to exercise competencies beyond dependency on mutual language expertise. One of the profound interactional consequences of these actions is redefining the default form of the brokering turn-taking system leading to restructuring the roles of participation. Many resources are found to aid the patients in constituting these forms of action initiation, some of which are the authority of experience, the overall structure of medical encounters, and the cognitive ability to monitor the ongoing interaction.

Action Initiation and the Authority of Experience

As language brokers re-reproduce—or, in Goffman's (1981) terms, animate—patients' talk, they occupy the interactional zone structurally sectioned for patients to convey their illness account, as exemplified in Excerpt (5). This fragment comes from a second visit to otolaryngologist office. Previously, the doctor prescribed a hearing-aid device, which the patient tried for over a month intolerably. In this visit, the patient returns with her son to correct the problem. Grammar mistakes in the script are original.

Excerpt (5): HAM: Hamid, son/language broker; SAL: Salma, patient

```
01     HAM:  the sound, it's not (0.3) very ||well.

02     SAL:                                   ||أبـــد.
02a                                           ||abad.
02b                                           ||not at all.

03     HAM:  even-even she adjust it. aah-

04     SAL:  وراسي يـوجعنـي مِن ||أحطها.
04a          wrāsi yūjaʿni min ||aḥu[ṭha.
04b          And my head hurts when ||I wear it.

05     HAM:                          ||دقـيقـة،
05a                                  ||minute,
05b                                  ||Wait a minute,

06     HAM:  even she adjust it, with the volume, but it's still the
07           sound, not hear it very well a::nd (.) she s::ay that, he=
08           =h:ad some headache o-on it.
```

The encounter begins with Hamid directly informing the doctor, rather than translating, about the purpose of the visit—that the sound of the device "is not very well." The agent in his sentence is the device or one of its properties. In line 2, Salma's voice comes to account for her condition as أبدا /abad/ [not at all/never]. Hamid, in line 05, treats her turn as an interruption and requests time to finish presenting her case. Passed the greeting, the encounter is still in the opening phase where the purpose of the visit is revealed to convey the reason behind using the medical time.

Understanding the structure of the medical visit has worked here as a resourceful object aiding the patient to execute her action (figure 3.1). The lexical /abad/ may appear to be an upgrade to Hamid's description. However, to consider an upgrading action, we must assume Salma's understanding of Hamid's prior turn, and that is unfeasible considering Salma's non-English

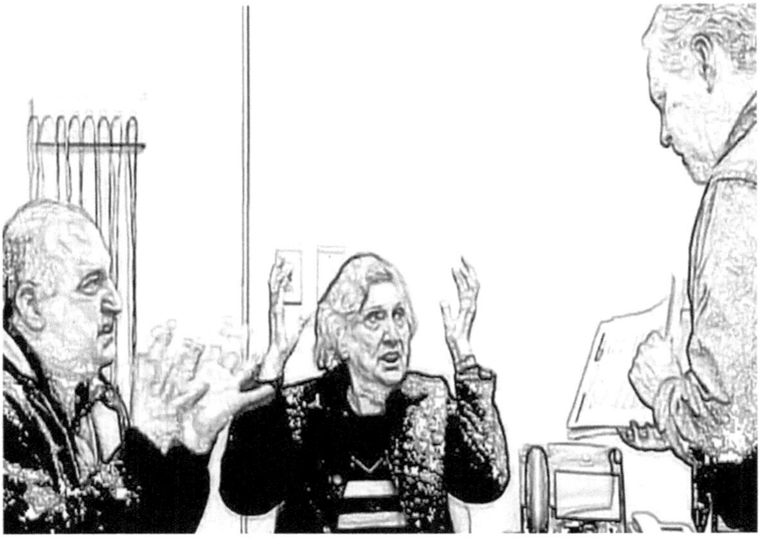

Figure 3.1 Hamid and Salma Describing the Medical Problem with Hands. *Source*: Author.

proficiency. Therefore, a different accountability has to explain Salma's action. Salma constructs her turn by recognizing her position as a patient with a primary epistemic right to tell her illness account (Heritage, 2012).

The progression of Hamid's and Salma's turns reveals their conflicting positions in regard to telling her case. Salma is the firsthand 'owner' of the experience, while Hamid is a 'witness' of the experience (Sacks, 1992). In line 04, Salma makes use of Hamid's hesitation in the prior turn, displayed by 'aah,' and proceeds to adds a second complaint that describes her head pain. She prefaces her turn with an *and*, arguing that these are two related issues. She presents herself as the agent reporting on her condition using first-person pronouns—"and my head hurts when I wear it." As the patient, Salma is the holder of her experience with the primary right to reveal its details. Through her turn, she argues that the central problem is located in her inability to hear and her headache (figure 3.3). Both complaints are equal and related medical conditions. Hamid starts his turn by describing the sound's quality (line 01) and continues from that point (line 06), saying that the sound is not good even if she adjusts it. But after Salma's turn, he switches from directly presenting the condition of the sound to reporting her medical condition of headaches by quoting her, "[S]he say [s] she had some headaches." He separates the illness account into two different problems: (1) the sound of the device and (2) headaches. Hamid's versus Salma's ways of launching the illness account are examples of imbalanced entitlement (Sacks, 1992; Heritage, 2012). Hamid learned about the condition from his mother; thus, his type of knowledge makes a difference in the manner of telling. Hamid's presentation reveals the malfunction of the device, but Salma's presentation shows that the medical conditions of not being able to hear and headaches are the reasons for the visits. Salma gives her account independently by recognizing her patienthood and the overall structure of the medical encounter.

Salma's delivery of her illness accounts forms a change in the brokering direction. Her interruption of her son's presentation changes the illness-telling sequence from direct communication, a language broker–doctor sequence, to a brokering communication of a language brokeree–language broker–doctor sequence so that a different pattern of interaction is constituted from the one started by Hamid. Hamid introduces himself as an immediate interlocutor reporting on a case within his type of knowledge, but his mother's initiation forces him to retreat and introduces the case from the point of her realm of knowledge as the direct owner of her experience. As such, Hamid retreats to transfer her words using the reported-speech code '[s]he say[s].'

Sacks notes, "[P]ersons who offer an account seem to feel that they're somehow committed to it, and if it turns out to be, for example, inadequate, then they have to stand by it" (Sacks, 1992, p. 5). Hamid commits to a position of presenting a case within his right to tell. When he switches to represent the case from her side, he uses a reporting code, saying "she says," and then qualifies her headaches by using a downgrading item as "*some* headaches" to embed himself as an evaluator of her condition. Their methods of presentation reveal different agendas: Hamid presents a technical account of a device; Salma presents a doctorable account of a medical condition.

Additionally, Salma uses Hamid's nonverbal communication as a contextual cue to construct her turn that overrides the brokering process. She monitors and builds her utterances as she analyzes the ongoing activity (figures 3.2 and 3.3).

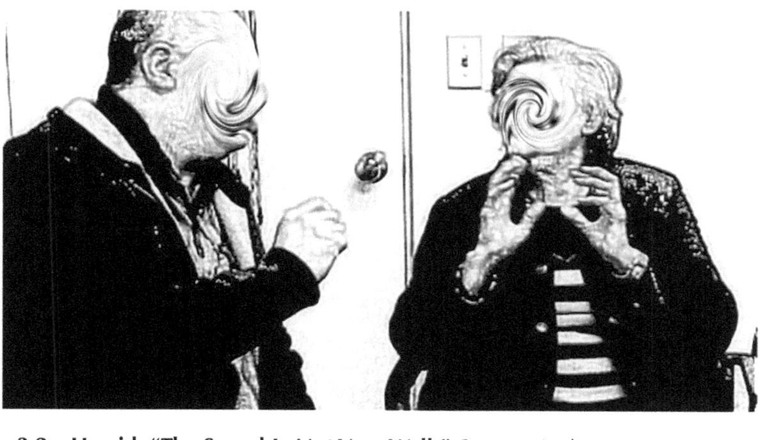

Figure 3.2 Hamid: "The Sound Is Not Very Well." *Source*: Author.

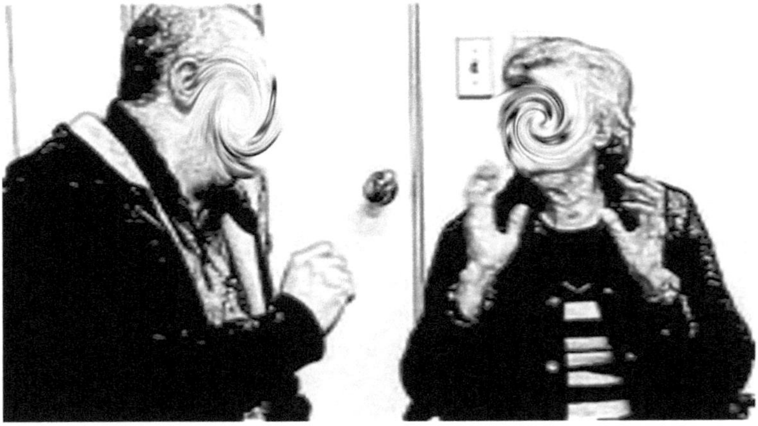

Figure 3.3 Salma: "And My Head Hurt When I Wear It." *Source*: Author.

Hamid talks to the doctor using hand gestures, while saying "the sound, it's not (0.3) very [well]," which worked as another contextual cue to inform Salma about the stage of ongoing talk as reaching a point of business, revealing the reason for the visit. His hand gesture, as in figure 3.2, resembles turning a nob of a device while his gaze is lowered. Salma looks at her son and starts shaping her hands to describe her head pain, as a sound wave hitting her head. In figure 3.3, she expresses that her head hurts while expanding her hands wider, physically and verbally demonstrating how she connects the sound quality with headaches. When hearing his mother's interference, Hamid lifts his eyes in recognition of her speech but requests to finish his turn. Salma uses the environment to inscribe herself in the conversation and gives her account without waiting for the interactional zone to be available. Salam responds to her son by building a nonverbal action occupying an interactional zone specifically sectioned to give a medical complaint. In doing so, she constitutes a form of unconventional initiated actions and redirects the LB turn-taking sequence to a default pattern. She builds her actions in Arabic, not mobilized by translation or direct solicitation from her broker or doctor.

As language brokerees are able to initiate actions independently (Jansson & Wadensjö, 2016), they are also able to respond to actions independently. They do so by closing the interactional space built for translation. Such turns do not represent sequentially initiated actions, but they constitute a form of initiation in the capacity of building actions independently. Through these actions, patients respond to the doctor's talk in English, showcasing their English competence. In other words, these actions do not fall in an initial position of FPP-2; nonetheless, they are acknowledged as initiations in the sense of being produced beyond the assistance of the LB order.

An example of this type of patients' deviant cases of initiation is displayed in the excerpt below. Karim (KAR), a seventy-three-year-old Iraqi man, visits a general practitioner with his son, Nathan (NAT), to seek help for a condition of fluid on his elbow collected due to a two-month-old injury. Karim has a modest capacity in English, limited to a few greetings and common small words, yet in the examples below, he performs complicated actions in English. Before seeing the doctor, a nurse took an X-ray of the injured area, filled out a medical history form, and then moved Karim and his son to a different room where the audio-recorded interaction below took place:

Excerpt (6): DOC: Doctor, NAT: Language broker, KAR: Patient

```
01   DOC:   Hell:o
02   NAT:   Hello doctor
03   DOC:   >Hi Hi<
04   NAT:   How are you?
05   DOC:   good it's Doctor Jenny nice to meet ya, nice to meet ya.
06   NAT:   nice to meet you doctor. how are you?
07   DOC:   good excellent let's switch those places, so who is the
08          patient?
09   KAR:   I am.
10   NAT:   mm abdul.
```

The medical interaction above opens with multiple sets of greetings exchanged between the language broker and the doctor. A noted quality of this opening is the multi-turns greeting sequence without the patient's participation. Greetings and "How are you" types of questions are interactional features of sociability (Heritage & Clayman, 2011), function as the beginning of the beginning (Sacks, 1992), and are often kept brief in institutional settings (Heritage & Drew 1992). The doctor opens the interaction with the first part of the greeting in line 1. Nathan, in line 2, greets back adding the word "doctor" that acts as a summon (Clayman, 2012), to which the doctor responds with a second greeting in a repetitive and rushed manner. In lines 04 and 05, and 06 and 07, the two exchange an additional two sets of greetings, initiated by Nathan. A greeting sequence is often followed by an introduction; thus, in line 05, the doctor answers Nathan quickly and proceeds to introduce himself formally greeting by introducing himself. The doctor then moves the conversation from a social to a medical exchange. In this lengthy dyadic exchange, Nathan inhibits the interactional floor and delays the doctor–patient conduct. Until now, and in Goffman's (1981) terms, the patient has been a *non-person* in a multiparty interaction and therefore enjoys a unique position to choose the entry slot into the conversation, as Karim does in line 09.

The sequence above is dominated by a dyadic exchange in which the language broker acts as a gatekeeper delaying the doctor–patient connection. In line 07, the doctor ends the greeting session and returns to business with the question "Who is the patient?" which serves as a switchboard request (Sidnell, 2010) to resume the interaction in the medical business after much delay. By design, questions are initiated actions that project a turn completing and therefore provide recipients with a resource to give a responsive action (Sacks, Schegloff, & Jefferson, 1974). In this question–answer sequence in lines 08 and 09, Karim seizes the opportunity offered to him by the doctor's tone and responds directly by closing the interactional floor for a translation turn. Although locationally, his turn falls in a sequence-responsive, rather than a sequence initiative, position; it is nevertheless the type of initiative considered here as a form of actuating patient's role and agency independently from the brokering process.

The issue we are after is how limited-English-speaking patients recognize and perform their patienthood in ways that transcend the brokering process to actuate an independent state of agency. This incident above exemplifies such actions. With an emphasis on the phrase 'I am,' Karim announces his role in the interaction as the patient, therefore the subject with the primary concern. His response, as provoked by the doctor's question, constitutes the direct alignment between him and his physician, who rearranges the seating's formation to bring Karim closer for an examination. Karim's direct response is also noted by Nathan who reclaims his role in line 10 and adds the first part of Karim's compound name, Abdul (a popular Arabic naming tradition, composed of double nouns, *abd*, the slave, or worshiper, plus one of the ninety-nine names of God as found in the Quran, prefaced with the definite article *al*, the; hence the compound name denotes the meaning "the God's worshiper"). Despite a novice level of English, Karim's response is initiated by understanding the patient's role, the projectivity of the question design, and by an intuitive need to be part of a conversation held on his account. Through the utility of these semiotic resources, he demonstrates his attentiveness to business/no-business parts of the conversation. His direct response to the doctor's question, while skipping an entrance into the prior greeting sequence, demonstrates a selective manner of interfering in the interaction and builds a direct channel of connecting with the doctor.

In the fragment below, the doctor examines Karim's arm. In line 52, he asks Karim about a sensation of numbness in his fingers. Despite novice English skills, Karim constructs an SPP-1, in which he responds to his doctor's question in English without translation. His response to this complicated question provokes an action of alignment by the doctor and an action of confirmation by the son, as shown below:

Excerpt (7):

```
44    DOC:   open your fingers.

45    NAT:   إفتح أصابيعك بابا،
45a          iftaḥ ʾaṣāby ʿak bāba,
45b          Open your fingers Dad,

             ((Karim spreads his fingers wide))

46    DOC:   try harder hardrr harrr,

47    NAT:   قوي قوي،
47a          gawi gawi,
47b          Harder Harder,

48    DOC:   very good.

49    NAT:   كلش زين.
49a          kuliš zeen.
49b          Very good.

50           (0.7)

51    DOC:   pain,

52    NAT:   ألم،
52a          ʾalam,
52b          pain,

53    KAR:   لا.
53a          lā.
53b          no.

54           (0.3)

55    DOC:   >°(okay)good<=
56           =↑no numbness or anything like [tha-
57    KAR:                                  [no no [no
58    DOC:                                         [oh oh oh
```

While the doctor holds Karim's hand to administrate an examination, Karim answers questions through brokering, forming the default sequence of the brokering discourse, FPP-1 FPP-R-2 SPP-2, constructed by the aid of nonverbal cues, followed by a sequence-closing turn in line 48, translated in line 49. Embedding verbal and nonverbal actions within the LB sequence, the doctor commands actions in lines 44 and 46, Nathen translates in lines 45 and 47, and Karim performs accordingly. In line 48, the doctor closes this sequence with an assessment token and starts another after a long pause. In line 52, another sequence begins where the three interlocutors coordinate another default LB sequence that concludes with a similar confirming token in a delayed but rushed manner (line 55). But in line 56, the doctor asks a question and Karim provides a direct response.

Enabled by several resources, Karim designs a turn without translation (line 57), as embedded in the handholding action. As the doctor holds the patient's hand, his question in line 56 invites a simple response to a 'no numbness' turn, directly following the question about the presence of pain in the earlier turn. In an overlap, Karim eliminates the transfer-relevance space for a translation turn and responds independently.

Karim builds an SPP-1 by performing an interactional competence referred to as *structure-preserving transformation*, in which a recipient unpacks a prior turn and preserves some of its parts to build the next turn (Goodwin, 2018). In line 55, the doctor utters *Okay* and *good* softly (as indicated by the degree marker), both are simple words and recognizable by Karim. He then marks *no* and *numbness* with stress on line 56. In line 57, Karim initiates a responsive action using the following resources: excluding simple words (okay, good, and nothing), preserving important words (no numbness), attending to a prior translated turn (the no-pain question), and acknowledging the nonverbal cue of hand-pressing. All these resources provide Karim with the opportunity to initiate his response in English independently despite the complicated doctor's question. Karim's ability to respond to this complex question got the attention of both his doctor and language broker. The doctor performs his next turn in line 58 in repetitive TCUs, matching Karim's turn in number and tone, while Nathan goes on multiple turns to confirm understanding, as shown below:

Excerpt (8):

```
60      NAT:    بـابـا يَعـنـي شِـنـو نـمـنس، تُعـرف؟
60a             bāba yaʿni šinū nummness, tʿruf?
60b             Dad what is numbness, do you know?

61      KAR:    أدري يـگـولـي أيـدك دَ دَ تـلـمس.
61a             adri, yguli eydak da da tlammas.
61b             I know, he tells me is is your hand tingling.

62      NAT:    لا- أي ي-يـعـنـي- أي.
62a             lā-ay y-yaʿni-ay.
62b             No-yes y-like-yes.

63      KAR:    يـعـنـي|| مـاكـو مـال هـيـچـي،
63a             yaʿni makū māl   ||hyği,
63b             Like something like this [way]

64      NAT:    ||تـنـمَل تـنـمَل
64a             ||tnamil||tnamil
64b             ||numb   ||numb
```

65 KAR: ||تنمل
65a ||tnamil
65b ||numb

66 NAT: مم تنمل اوكي.
66a mm tnamil ūkay
66b mm numb okay

67 KAR: أي، هذا لي أقصده.
67a ay, haḏa li-aquṣda.
67b Yeah, that it's what I mean.

Between lines 60 and 67, Nathan initiates a multiple-turn sequence to confirm his father's understanding, but in essence, he is also confirming his language-broker position. The item ماكو makū is a common Iraqi negative phrase that serves many functions one which denotes an action of resemblance by suggesting a process of eliminating possibilities. In line 63, the father seems to enact his understanding of the word 'numbness,' as saying 'like this.' Still, the son takes a few turns before acknowledging that his father indeed has provided the correct response. In this example, the patient constructs an action that constitutes immediate conduct with his physician, thus avoiding the proxy of brokering and redirecting the discourse, if momentarily, to a dyadic doctor–patient interaction.

Combating a Forced Identity

Sometimes, a membership category is assigned or assumed by others. In this section, we discuss a case in which the mother ascribes the language brokeree's identity to her adolescent son who speaks English comfortably. Continuing with her ways of managing the family's affairs, the mother depends on her oldest daughter to facilitate family needs with the outside world. Although some of her kids have grown more comfortable with English, the mother continues to navigate her outside responsibilities by soliciting the help of her oldest daughter, Nada. Nada is a seventeen-year-old high-school student and the family's designated language broker from El Cajon, San Diego.

The purpose of this visit is to check on Selim's wrist. Selim is a fourteen-year-old boy, the only son in a family of four children. Earlier that month, he fell during a soccer game and fractured his right wrist. During this visit, Selim's cast, which he received three weeks earlier in the local hospital, was removed and an X-ray was taken before meeting the doctor. Selim, his mother, two sisters, the language broker, and the baby sister were present at the doctor's office. The visit lasted 3 minutes and 40 seconds. The fragment below starts with Selim explaining the accident to the doctor. Before that, the language broker, Nada, announced that she would be translating for her mother. As Nada tries to explain the purpose of the visit (un-transcribed), Selim grabs the interactional floor to tell his experience (line 1 below). At the beginning of this interaction, the doctor directs his question, gaze, and body position toward the mother, who in turn looks at Nada for interpretation. Selim redefines his doctor–patient relationship by presenting himself as an immediate interlocutor:

Excerpt (9): SEL: Selim/patient, NAD: Nada, sister/language broker, DOC: Doctor

```
01   SEL:  ahh I wz playing soccer and I fell on it.
02   DOC:  Okay (0.1) and this wa::s January first?=
03   SEL:  =January first ((with a head node))
04         (0.1)
05   DOC:  Okay ((writing down on his chart))
06   SEL:  °>first day of NBA< ((smiling))
07   DOC:  okay (0.2) th:en w-was he seen here, or where's seen=
08         he seen=
           ((Shifting his gaze between the mother and the
             daughter))
09   SEL:  =Yeah I was seen here.
10   NAD:  in [the emergency room ((The doctor turns to look
           at Selim))
11   SEL:     [at the emergency room.
12   DOC:  okay,
```

Children's participation in medical visits is often promoted by doctors' questions that are found to involve children as young as two-and-a-half years old. Traditionally, however, doctors gather needed information from parents, sometimes even when the patient child is around ten years old or older (Stivers & Majid, 2007). Though Selim is fourteen years old and has demonstrated his language ability in lines 01, 03, and 06, the doctor, perhaps in response to the earlier announcement of the presence of a conversation mediator, solicits information from the mother, who in turn gazes toward her daughter for translation. Selim redefines his relationship with his doctor by grabbing turns through which he insists on giving his account. In this excerpt, Selim redefines this child patient–physician relationship and simultaneously discredits his language brokeree's status. He demonstrates his linguistic skills through his ability to provide his own medical account directly. In line 01, Selim answers the doctor's question about the cause of the accident, and in line 03, he confirms the doctor's information by a partial repetition of the doctor's prior utterance indexing an independent state of knowing (Heritage & Raymond, 2005). Once the information is received, the doctor closes the sequence with an 'okay' in line 05, but Selim solicits a rapport with the doctor (line 06), adding that the accident coincided with the start of the NBA, the national basketball tournament (although it might have been just a specific game as the regular NBA season often starts earlier). The next question is also directed toward the mother. In lines 07 and

08, the doctor asks about the place of the first treatment. Even though the doctor's body orientation is directed toward the mother, Selim performs a self-selected turn by latching his response to the doctor's prior utterance reporting on the location where he was admitted (line 09). His sister takes the floor to specify that the 'here' refers to the emergency room of the same hospital where this interaction takes place. Selim again rushes to confirm his right to tell his experience and affirms his English competence by overriding his sister's talk.

In this episode, the identity of a language brokeree is assigned by the mother rather than mandated by the son's language ability, but the son challenges the ascribed role by asserting his independent state of patienthood.

CONCLUSION

In this chapter, I revisited the interactional accomplishments of language brokerees by focusing specifically on the organization of initiated actions. Two forms of action initiation were located: a default conventional form, and deviant unconventional form. The default form occupies the first part of a sequence and performed mostly in Arabic to request a recap of previously given information, add extra complaints, and ask about important details of upcoming treatment steps. On several occasions, these initiatives are hampered from developing into triadic LB sequences when treated with silence or answered directly without engaging the doctor.

The second type of action initiation is formed by overriding the brokering process to actuate an independent state of patienthood. Actions of this type fall in a responsive position, forming examples of a deviant case of initiation based on the fact that they constitute a direct doctor–patient exchange and by activating an independent state of involvement. They display a simple, yet contextually appropriate, bilingual competency. They signify the enactment of human cognition and sociability in challenging environments.

Interactionally, these involvements redefine the structure of brokering turn-taking systems so that patterns of participation are also restructured. They change the default triadic sequence of doctor–language broke–patient, or patient–language broker–doctor, to a dyadic sequence of a direct patient–doctor conduct. Sometimes, patients' actions restore a triadic exchange from a doctor–language broker sequence to a patient–language broker–doctor sequence to deliver their account through the language-assistance turn. Language-brokering and interpretation scholarships have studied the nonnormative turn-taking sequence, focusing on the actions of language brokers and professional interpreters. This chapter shows normative and nonnormative turn-taking systems performed based on the language brokerees' initiatives in which patients challenge contextual asymmetries inherent in their brokered interactions. In doing so, they contradict the stereotypical way of perceiving limited-English-speaking patients as interactants via the proxy of brokering only. The brokering process is indeed essential in crosslinguistic encounters. The analyses in this chapter are not aimed to discount the language brokers' efforts but to foreground the actions of the language brokeree within the language-brokering activity as essential to meaning-making.

Chapter 4

Asserting Patienthood through Expansion

This chapter expands our examination of patients' agency by exploring another sequential organization of action initiation. It specifically focuses on cases in which the Iraqi patients in this study organize actions by extending prior turns voluntarily. The interactional position where such actions become possible is identified as post-sequence expansion. Patients insert their input to correct wrong information, assess when language discordance emerges, and request inclusion in the business/no-business parts of their medical encounters. In such cases, monitoring the interaction in English works as nonverbal cues, employed resourcefully as operative sequences upon which patients build their next turns. This chapter robustly demonstrates the interactional affordances provided by the post-sequence position. Analyses show how the epistemological authority underscores volunteered engagement so that personal investments and human agency are interactionally interplayed.

In the previous chapter, we discussed how limited-English-speaking patients influence the LB turn-taking system based on initiatives motivated mostly by exercising their speakership right as the owners of their illness experiences. They activate multiple social membership categories fluidly as patients, parents, and language brokerees by exploring available environmental semiotic resources, including the structure of medical visits and their linguistic abilities. Through their own initiatives, they interact cooperatively with and independent from the brokering process, the organization of their actions influences visits' turn-taking system so that patterns of participation are also altered

The analyses in this chapter feature post-sequence expansion as another sequential locus for studying the constitution of patients' agency through which their interactional competency and personal investment emerge visibly. These turns operate on the structure of adjacency pair to offer relatable actions.

They accomplish various important actions, some of which are affirming visits' agenda, clarifying erroneous information, and aiding language brokers as needed. Patients form these actions voluntarily, without physicians' or language brokers' involvement, further sustaining their engagement in all parts of their medical visits. Recognizing actions in this position demonstrates that attending to limited-English-speaking patients' interactional contributions must be sustained throughout the encounter, not specific to a certain medical phase.

SEQUENCE EXPANSION

Although social actions are systematically defined in terms of adjacency pairs, their projected interactional agenda in a given setting is hardly accomplished within a singular pair of FPP and SPP. For example, preferred actions are found to be performed without mitigation or delay (Pomerantz, 1984), while discordant actions are designed with some form of mitigation (Clayman, 2002). These interactional mechanisms are studied as examples of constructing agreement and disagreement (Pomerantz, 1984), authority and entitlement (Heritage, 2002; Sacks, 1992), identity (Raymond et al., 2021), among others. Although these actions could be achieved in one or more unites of adjacency pairs, their extended work is normatively examined as part of the base pair, rather than as separate phenomena patients, creating forms of inclusions to give them an entry into closely structured conversations (Jansson & Wadnesjö, 2016).

Schegloff (2007) identifies extended actions that operate on the base adjacency pair in three sequential locations: pre-sequence, insert sequence, and post-sequence. He argues that all adjacency pairs are potentially open for expansion. In regard to post-sequence expansion, he categorizes two types—minimal and nonminimal expansions—and identifies several types of each. The minimal post-sequence expansion is mostly constructed to project closing. By design, they offer no further comment on the topic for which the base adjacency pair was formed. The achievements of small talk have received a fair amount of attention among CA scholars, such as the use of "Okay" among doctors, as in the broken-wrist episode we have seen in the previous chapter.

Excerpt (1):

```
SEL: →  ahh I wz playing soccer and I fell on it.
DOC:    Okay (0.1) and this wa::s January first?=
SEL:    =January first ((with a head node))
        (0.1)
DOC:    Okay ((writing down on his chart))
```

In line 01, Selim explains that he fell and broke his wrist while playing soccer; upon receiving this information, the doctor asks another question about the accident's time. In both cases, the doctor closes the question–answer sequence with an "Okay," in lines 02 and 05, to move forward.

The second form of sequence expansion is identified as a nonminimal expansion. Such turns are built with more than one item of utterances and can often invite follow-up turns to open the base sequence. Recent work has explored how the position of post-sequence expansion is utilized in educational contexts as a resource to manage topic development and patterns of participation. Jacknick (2011) examines ESL education and notes that students expand on teachers' questions and comments to redirect class discussions in ways that allow them to influence their own learning experiences and challenge teachers' authority about the distribution of knowledge and participatory roles. Expanding on this line of research, this chapter explores the utility of the post-sequence expansion in mobilizing the agency of limited-English-speaking patients.

The history-taking medical phase is said to progress according to the doctor's agenda in pursuit of a certain medical hypothesis, in which accuracy is supported or dismissed by patients' answers (Boyd & Heritage, 2006). In the examined data, this part of brokered medical encounters appears to be dominated by the language brokers' answers, as exemplified in the fragment below.

Excerpt (2):

```
82    DOC:   any medical problems,

83    NAT:   عِندك مَشاكِل صحيّة،
83a          ʿindak mašākil ṣḥiyya,
83b          Do you have medical problems,

84    KAR:   بـــ||س-
84a          b||es-
84b          j||ust-

85    NAT:   ||ha-high blood pressure. Diabetes=
86    DOC:   =diabetes?
87    NAT:   a::nd cholesterol.

88    KAR:   كَليسترول. (٠.١) يعني بَس-
88a          kalistrōl. (0.1) yaʿni bes-
88b          cholesterol. (0.1) Like just-

89    DOC:   on-on mm insulin or no insulin,
90    NAT:   no insulin, just pills.
```

In line 82, the doctor asks about the patient's medical history. Nathan translates first in line 83 but quickly abandons his role as a language broker and chooses to answer directly, and in doing so, he contributes to an already tardy connection between the doctor and this patient due to lacking mutual intelligibility (lines 85, 87, & 90). In lines 84 and 88, the patient tries to participate, but he gets interrupted by his son's direct response to the doctor's question. In line 86, the doctor repeats an item from the prior turn that gets his attention, but his seeking-information uptake fails to stop the language broker who continues to list other medical problems. The patient picks on a familiar word—cholesterol—a borrowed item in Arabic and tries to add his account in line 88. The doctor grabs another turn in line 89 to request information about the patient's diabetes, asking whether insulin is used to treat his condition; the request is also answered by the language broker. The interaction here is expanded beyond the initial question/answer base sequence in an attempt to collect required pieces of information. As apparent, this sequentially built resource is occupied by participants as an interactional tool to coordinate information transferring and access to participation. The language broker holds the interactional floor to claim his right to immediate speakership, while the doctor and the patient add their own input to correct or complete the patients' medical story. At this point, the language broker acts as a gatekeeper managing the passing of information and the distribution of roles.

Later in the above visit during the examination phase, Karim responds to a doctor's question independently, as shown elsewhere. Nathen builds many questions to check for understanding, as shown below:

Excerpt (3):

```
60      NAT:  بابا يَعني شنِو نمنس، تُعرف؟
60a           bāba yaʿni šinū numbness, tʿruf?
60b           Dad what is numbness, do you know?

61      KAR:  أدري يگولي أيدك دَ دَ تلمس.
61a           adri, yguli eydak da da tlammas.
61b           I know, he tells me is is your hand tingling.

62      NAT:  لا-أي ي-يعني-أي.
62a           lā-ay y-yaʿni-ay.
62b           no-yes y-like-yes.

63      KAR:  يعني ماكو مال ||هيچي,
63a           yaʿni makū māl ||hyği,
63b           Like something like this [way]

64      NAT:  ||تنمَل تنمَل
64a           ||tnamil ||tnamil
64b           ||numb   ||numb

65      KAR:  ||تنمَل
65a           ||tnamil
65b           ||numb

66      NAT:  ممـ تنمَل، أوكي.
```

```
66a          mm tnamil ūkay
66b          mm numb okay

67    KAR:   أي، هذا لي اقْصده.
67a          ay, haḏa li-aquṣda.
67b          Yes, that it's what I mean.
```

In line 60, Nathen produces a confirmation check to make sure that his father has understood and responded to the right issue. In line 61, the father proves that he indeed has understood the doctor's question and answered accordingly. Nevertheless, Nathen posts multiple question–answer sequences to confirm understanding(lines 62–66), through which he also affirms his position as the manager of the information-passing dynamic, which was violated by Karim's direct response. This is especially clear in line 62, "لا-أي ي يعني-أي" [no-yes y like-yes]. The TCUs here form the following actions: denial (لا/no), acknowledgment (أي/yes), hesitation (ي/y), interjection (يعني/like [meaning]), another acknowledgment (أي/yes). This multiple-TCUs turn enfolds various actions to reluctantly give the green light about Karim's understanding of the doctor's complicated question. Both the language broker and the language brokeree hold the confirmation-checking sequence so that they mutually demonstrate their knowledge and competence, finally arriving at an agreement that the correct answer was given. Although both speakers have asserted their interactional roles, Karim closes the sequence by affirming his speakership's right and his English competence in a nonminimum post-sequence closing turn, as saying "yeah, that's what I mean."

The position of post-sequence expansion operates in this example as a zone of confirming contextual roles for both Karim an Nathan. They tightly claim their authoritative membership categories so that Karim affirms his patienthood and in situ English competence and Nathan affirms his conversation-coordinating role. The contextual negotiation of abilities and identities leans toward Karim, as he takes that last turn to confirm his sound understanding and ability to respond. The rest of this chapter will focus on analyzing the functions of actions in the post-sequence-expansion position, centering on patients' agendas.

PATIENTS' EXPANSIONS

Observing the organization of post-sequence expansion further foreshows the unabating attention patients exercise when managing their healthcare within the constraints imposed by discursive brokering and institutional norms. Patients' exploitation of this interactional position functions to serve their patient agendas in the manner of actuating contextual identities, clarifying translation errors, and mending meaning-making when misunderstandings emerge

In the example below, Selim, the teenager with the broken wrist, responds to the doctor's question about the bruise on his wrist. Selim answers and then expands to pursue a personal agenda, as noted below. (Grammar mistakes in Selim's turns are original.)

Excerpt (4):

```
53   DOC:  and that doesn't hurt though?
54   SEL:  no=
55   DOC:  =this (0.1) bruising ha:s been since the injury?
56   SEL:  Yeah,
57   DOC:  okay.
58   SEL:  but it's (.0) a lot more. like it waz from he::re to here,
59         and it was more darker it was a::ll purple.
60   DOC:  Okay okay, so it is better now?
61   SEL:  Yeah it doesn't hurt.
```

The evaluation of Selim's pain in line 53 is formulated through a question designed as negatively polarized declarative to facilitate a no-type response by: 1- affirming the negative statement "that doesn't hurt," and then 2- tailoring it with "though." The projectivity of confirming a negative state of pain is specially enhanced with "and," as a conclusive item. Although the doctor offers Selim a chance to confirm a desired no-pain condition, tailing his turn with "though" suggests a level of discrepancy between the two in defining pain. In line 54, Selim denies feeling pain in the injured area with his short and direct token of denial, 'no.' His confident response is challenged by the doctor who associates the existence of the dark-purple bruised area with a sustained injury. In line 55, the doctor designs his question to project a "best-guess" scenario (Heritage, 2010). Selim's response, "Yeah," suffices to close the sequence with an "Okay." *Okays* are the type of items that function as a disjunction between previous and upcoming topics (Beach, 1995, 2020; Heritage, 1984; Jefferson, 1978). Selim, however, halts the project of moving forward. In line 58, Selim initiates an unsolicited post-sequence expansion turn to account for the doctor's possible reluctance to associate the purple area with signs of recovery, as tacitly suggested by Selim's description of a shrinking-color zone. He designs a rather effortful turn with multiple TCUs to explain a recovery process unwitnessed by the doctor; the purple area was wider and darker than how it looks now under the doctor's viewing. By suggesting a vanishing bodily witness, Selim attempts to convince the doctor that his arm is recovering, even though it still looks purple (figure 4.1). His project is visible in the way he organizes his turn through these structures: a qualifier (a lot), an intensifier (more), verbal and nonverbal measuring actions (here

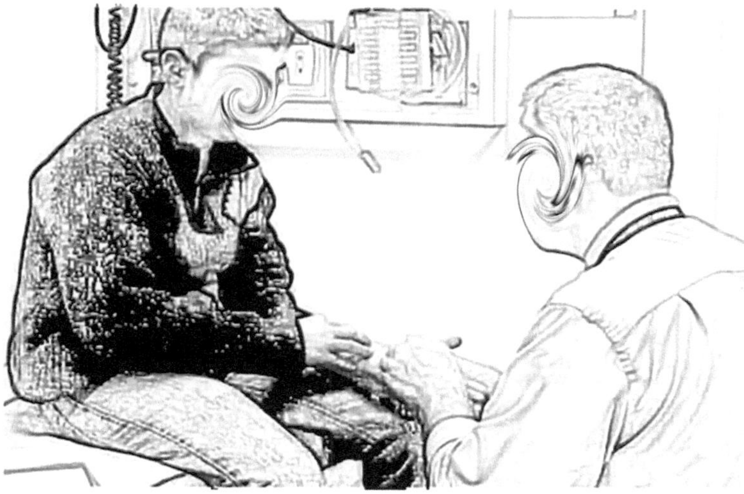

Figure 4.1 Selim: "It Was From Here to Here, and It Was More Darker, It Was All Purple." *Source:* Author.

to here with passing his hand on the purple area on his arm), a comparative items (darker), another descriptive qualifier (all purple), and a vowel lengthening (h::r, a::ll), quite an effort and effective exploitation of grammatical items for a new language user.

On line 60, the doctor acknowledges Selim's efforts with (1) repetitive tokens of agreement, (2) a conclusive item, "so," foreshadowing an upcoming evaluation, and (3) a declarative assessment verbalized in a question tone, "It's better now?," giving Selim the authority of confirming a final conclusion. The doctor designs an action-based preference for confirmation in which he transfers the primacy of judgment to the patient (Heritage & Sefi, 1992). According to Selim, it is not just better, the broken wrist does not hurt anymore (line 61). Although the doctor and the patient have worked on opposite ways of assessing the injured area, one by building a case of a sustained bruise and another by building a case of a recovering bruise, they both worked their way to reach a final agreement. The mother understands Selim's project. She later cleared that Selim loves soccer and he has missed his high-school season because of his injury; thus, he wishes to receive the doctor's clearance to resume playing (un-transcribed). These actions are afforded by the effective utility of post-sequence expansion.

In the interaction below, the doctor arranges the seating to bring the patient closer in order to perform a medical examination. In line 12, and with an overlap, the patient initiates an unsolicited post-sequence expansion to the seating arrangement, which works here as an introductory-sequence completion of an earlier action. In line 09, Karim identifies his role as the patient; the doctor's identity and name have been established earlier. In line 12, Karim clears his relation to Nathen, as saying ‘my son,’ thus completing an earlier halted introductory segment:

Excerpt (5):

```
09     NAT:    mm ab[dul.
10     DOC:          [okay you sit there you've a [seat here,
11     KAR:                                       [my son.
12     DOC:    and I'll sit here and now we're all comfortable.
```

The doctor has exchanged multiple turns of greetings with the language broker (examined elsewhere), without identifying his role or relation to the patient. His concern is identifying the patient so that the medical business begins. Karim initiates a delayed post-sequence turn to an incomplete introductory action. After responding to the question that identifies his role, he gives an unsolicited explanation to identify the third interlocutor, “my son,” in line 11.

In the excerpt below, the doctor asks about the medical drugs Karim currently takes. As a caregiver and a family member, Nathen feels he has the information to answer directly. Yet, when Karim receives the translation, he adds more materials through which he sustains an active involvement, the type of information that is usually owned by the owner of the medical experience, the patient:

Excerpt (6):

```
90     DOC:   on- on mm insulin or no insulin,
91     NAT:   no insulin, just pills.

92     NAT:   بس مَـــ||اتـاخُذ حبـايـة، مَتـاخُذ أنـسولـيـن,
92a           bes tāxuḏ ḥabāya, ma||tāxuḏ insūlyn,
92b           You just take a pill, you don'ta||take insulin,

93     KAR:   ||no no
94            (0.2)

95            وبـس حبـايـة. ونص، مـيـتـيـن وخـمـسـيـن.
95a           wbes ḥabāya. wnuṣ, myten wxamsyn.
95b           And just a pill, and a half, two hundred fifty.

96     NAT:   okay okay two hundred fifty.
97     DOC:   okay.
```

The doctor requests information on the diabetic condition (line 90); Nathan responds directly (line 91) and then retracts to request a validation of his given answer (line 92). Interpretation studies have noted the prevalence of this type of backchannel translation in causal and professional contexts

(Wadensjö, 2014), which invalidates the advantage of receiving immediate answers, although they might be wrongly understood and favored by doctors on the merits of saving times (Davidson, 1998, 2001). The language brokerees, as noted thus far, act within the constraints imposed on their participation to manage and direct interactions toward serving their patient's agenda. Here, Karim takes the interactional floor to make his voice heard, as in line 95 by specifying the dosage of his medicine. In this action, Karim explicates his speakership by providing unsolicited information, adding that his condition is indeed managed by pills and only half of the regular dosage, /wnuṣ/ [and half]. By specifying the quantity of his medicine prefaced with an "and," Karim asserts the manageability of his condition and sustains his right to tell it. He distinguishes his type of knowledge, an owner of an experience, from the broker's knowledge, an observer of an experience.

Sometimes, patients' actions reveal important misunderstandings due to wrong translation. An example of such situations comes from Salma, the patient with hearing problems. Salma keenly monitors the ongoing interaction and perform relevant actions when needed, especially when Hamid seems to struggle with his fluency. In the segment below, Salma's interference reveals a gap between the requested and received information, as exemplified below:

Excerpt (7):

```
165     DOC:    have she ever had a loud noise exposure?
166     HAM:    loud noise?
167     DOC:    ve she ever been around-like in a job where there's
168             real loud- a lot or there-ahh-

169     HAM:    تسمَعين فد أصوات قويّة، فد شي مِن مِن-آه ه
169a            tsmaʿyn fad āṣwat qawiyya fad ši min min-ahh
169b            Do you hear strong sounds, something from from-ahh

170     SAL:    .لا
170a            lā.
170b            No.

171     HAM:    no, she doesn't.
172     DOC:    okay.
173             (0.2)

174     SAL:    بس ما-مَف-مَاسمع التلفزيون.
174a            ((Extending her hand at the distance)) bes ma-maf-
                  masmaʿ ltalfzyūn.
174b            I just don't-und-I don't hear the TV.
```

The above fragment is part of the history-taking phase, when the doctor asks if Salma has been exposed to surrounding load noises. His question is transferred as a question about a current situation, if she hears strong voice (Hamid uses *strong* instead of *loud*, but both adjectives could be used interchangeably when describing the quality as being noisy or disruptive). The doctor's question specifies an external and old environment, but the translation suggests an internal and current condition. Salma denies that she hears sounds and then adds that she is just unable to hear the TV, extending her arm to metaphorically depict the distance between her seating and the TV. In line 166, Hamid repeats the utterance "load noise," indicating a trouble with understanding (Drew, 1997), to which the doctor responds with repetition and examples, but shows a difficulty of coming up with more helping descriptions (doctors are certainly not trained to mend language barriers). Hamid's repetition of (min min) is followed by a breathing sound 'ahh' reflecting a continuous difficulty with providing suitable translation. Salma's answer in line 170 merely negates the question, but her expansion (line 74) makes it analytically visible that the doctor has received the wrong information.

Expansion as an Action of Reversed Brokering

As language brokers offer their time and expertise to assess family members, they themselves might struggle with the dominant language and culture or the heritage language and culture. On such occasions, the language brokerees reclaim their parenting role and come to the aid of their helpers. In the excerpt below, the language broker, repeatedly, also expectedly, transgresses his interpreting duties to give the required information. In line 184, he performs a few false starts before completing his sentence. In line 187, his mother, the patient Salma, comes to help him in a turn that achieves several actions, as will be explained:

Excerpt (8):

181 DOC: all the med she's taking right now?
((Extending a form to Hamid))
182 HAM: yes, this one for-for thi:s time-
183 DOC: okay.
184 HAM: because she has some-some p-pro-problem with ahh with am
185 bl||ood pressure.
186 DOC: okay.

187 SAL: ||هاي مال ضغط؟
187a ||hāi māl ḍaǧuṭ?
187b ||This for the blood pressure?

```
188     HAM:  أي هـوَ ذيـگولـي،
188a          ay hwa dayqūli
188b          Yes, he's saying that to me,
```

In line 181, the doctor asks about Salma's medicine by extending a form he holds in his hand. He directs the form, his gaze, and a question to Hamid, while referring to Salma as *she*. The question–answer sequence in lines 181 and 182 are a dyadic exchange about a third party who is present but treated priori as absent. Through these actions, the doctor selects to treat Hamid as his primary interlocutor. Upon receiving the answer, the doctor attempts to close the sequence (line 183), but Hamid rejects the doctor's project through multiple restarts and repairs to explain that the medicine on the form is for her blood-pressure condition. Goodwin and Goodwin (1986) note that if a participant has difficulty finding a word, other conversation participants often provide a candidate response to progress the talk. Salma recognizes Hamid's efforts and offers unsolicited assistance, achieved by monitoring her interlocutors' nonverbal actions. When the doctor asks Hamid in line 181, he leans forward to show the form, making it visible in Salma's vision field. Salma, sitting between the doctor and Hamid, recognizes the form that they filled with the nurse before meeting the doctor. As she notices her son's visible effort in finishing his utterances, Salma overlaps with her son and constructs an Arabic turn, stating that the listed medicine is for her blood pressure (line 187). Both Hamid and Salma coordinate bilingual post-sequence-expansion turns to provide the needed information.

Salma's volunteered post-sequence expansion is mobilized by interpreting the nonverbal actions of her conversation partners: the doctor's extended arm with the form and Hamid's effortful turn to finish his sentence. She performs her turn with a high-raising tone verbalized softly, suggesting an implicit action of soliciting confirmation. She verbalizes her utterances with a soft voice possibly to avoid further marking her son's arduous efforts visible (Brown & Levinson, 1987). This Arabic post-sequence expansion is accomplished by monitoring the ongoing activity through which Salma sustains involvement during unintelligible parts of the conversation.

Salma's initiated actions demonstrate an agentive enactment of her attentiveness to the progressivity of her medical interaction. Through her unsolicited actions, Salma embeds herself as an active and equal partner in the meaning-making process. In the example below, Salma and her son visit an eye doctor as a post-surgery checkup. Salma had a cataract surgery on her right eye a week before the meeting of the fragment below. In this visit, Salma and Hamid see the nurse first:

Excerpt (9): HAM: Hamid/son, Nur: Nurse, SAL: Salma/patient

```
28   HAM:  .hh because we've some ahhh mm-un-.hh understood I=
29         =between the pharm:acy and between the doctor about=
30         = what they said.
31   NUR:  okay, ||need to be-
32   HAM:  ahhh that way we||need to be-

33   SAL:  ||شوف-اكو ورقة من الطبيب.
33a        ||shūf-akū wraqa min lṭabyb.
33b        ||Look-there is a paper from the doctor.

34   HAM:  >yeah yeah<                   ((to his mother))
35         we need to be clear on it,     ((to the nurse))
36   NUR:  sure, no problem.
37         (0.3)              ((Hamid unfolds a paper))
38   HAM:  this what the pharmacy write. and this what the doctor-
39         (0.1) he give us a description about the drops so we just=
40         =need to be sure of ahh this kind which one.
41   NUR:  Okay.=
42   HAM:  =okay,
```

In the excerpt above, Hamid explains with some difficulty that there is a discrepancy between the doctor's instructions and the information they received from the pharmacist. On lines 28–30, he initiates many false starts and repairs to finish his sentence, while holding a medicine bottle and pointing to the label. Salma notices his efforts to complete his sentence and comes to his help. In line 33, she directs him to find a paper that explains the situation better, which Hamid acknowledges by a rushed, double-token confirmation, "yeah, yeah." In lines 43 and 44, he explains the situation, while holding the note he found as instructed by his mother. Thus far, Hamid has taken care of the nurse encounter on his own. However, Salma's attentiveness to the interaction, though in English, worked in the capacity of nonlinguistic cues to affirm her inclusion in the conversation.

Requests for Inclusion

While taking care of business, doctors are encouraged to develop social rapport with their patients. In the excerpt below, which we have met elsewhere, the doctor asks about the circumstance of the injury. The patient responds by confirming the doctor's information found on the patient's chart but continues to give a nonmedical comment.

Excerpt (10):

```
01   SEL:   ahh I wz playing soccer and I fell on it.
02   DOC:   Okay (0.1) and this wa::s January first?=
03   SEL:   =January first.        ((with a head node))
04          (0.1)
05   DOC:   Okay                   ((writing down on his chart))
06   SEL:   °>first day of NBA< ((smiling))
07   DOC:   okay
```

Selim confirms the doctor's information on the time of the incident and then adds a life-event recording of his injury. His action is met by the doctor with the common "okay," denying an implicit invitation to engage in a nonmedical exchange.

A similar call for inclusion comes from Salma (see below). Thus far, we have witnessed Salma effortfully work to take part in her medical interactions throughout different phases of her medical encounters. In the fragment below, she also agentively requests to be included in the nonmedical part of the interaction.

Excerpt (11):

```
193    DOC:  and you don't know of any family history of
194          hearing loss. Right?
195    HAM:  I'm her son. [(.) so haha we don't have any [hahahah
196    DOC:              [hah    hhaa
197    HAM:              [no family
198          history of hearing loss. only onl||y-her-

199    SAL:                                          ||شِنو؟
199a                                                 ||šinū?
199b                                                 ||What?

200    HAM:  يـگول عِدكُم أحد بِالعائِلة مَيسمع،
200a         yqūl ʿidkum āḥd bilʿāʾila maysmaʿ,
200b         He said do you have someone in the family who
             doesn't hear,
```

The question about the family health history is polarized by a triple-type grammatical composition: 1- A preposition about a state of knowing designed in a negative declarative "you don't know," 2- a postulation of a solid state of knowing through "any," and 3- an invitation to confirm the two proposals by a tag question, "right?" The doctor's method of fishing for the desired information requests a double-form affirmation: 1- affirming the assumption he made about Hamid's knowledge, and 2- affirming a moral ground upon which the question was posted to Hamid. Ultimately, the doctor negotiates Hamid's primacy to reveal the family background (Heritage, 2012; Heritage & Clayman, 2010). The probability of Hamid's knowledge about an existence of hearing problem in his lineage is not an unreasonable one, considering his age level being in mid-fifties. However, even though Hamid might have access to such information, Salma is the immediate owner of the hearing-loss experience. Her primacy to respond to the question is also built on two accounts: being an older family member, and being a sufferer of the condition. The utility of the considerably involved grammatical structure to request a common type of information underpins the doctor's tacit orientation toward the sensitive topic of speakership rights. The language barrier prevents the doctor from providing Salma the right to tell her own medical narrative. In lines 195-198, Hamid confirms the likelihood of knowing his family background and addresses the doctor's tacit suspicion through a laughter. Both the doctor and Hamid join in laughter recognizing the potential vulnerability of the question. Salma has been excluded from this exchange until she explicitly demands to be included. She requests an explanation by asking شِنو؟, /šinū/ [What?]. Her minimally designed question is afforded by observing the laughter to implicitly requesting her presence to be acknowledged in the no-business episode. Salma's inclusion in this episode is generated only by attending to the English dyadic exchange and the laughter that worked as nonverbal resources to furnish Salma's turn in a post-sequence position.

CONCLUSION

This chapter deals with a specific sequential property of the brokering medical turn-taking system, the position of post-sequence expansion. The analyses demonstrate how interlocutors actuate their state of knowledge that endows them with the content and right to talk. They play an agentive role, in which they claim their multiple identities as a language broker—by requesting translation when it is absent, as a patient—by supplying necessary information even when their involvement is not directly solicited, and as a parent—by helping their language brokers to mend linguistic and informational gaps. These actions are voluntarily produced to supply relevant inputs mobilized by keen observation of the English interactions, which effectively act as contextual nonlinguistic cues.

These findings affirm another vital aspect of the active commitment of limited-English-speaking patient. They demonstrate their ability to embed themselves in the interaction as cognitive and social actors beyond the default sequential spots for patients' contributions in the forms of initiating actions or providing answers. In the previous chapter, we found that our patients build actions and responses by operating on many semiotic resources. They also close the relevant transitional floor for translation to offer their own responses independently. In this chapter, our patients build actions even when actions are not formed as question/answer sequences, which are said to occupy about 80 percent of the doctor–patient encounters. They also act when their participation is not sought and when the conversation is in English. They proactively exploit the sequential organization of the brokering turn-taking system, here in the post-sequence-expansion position, to fashion participation that is often not solicited or accounted for. In so doing, they effectively constitute their multiple social membership categories as patients, language brokerees, and parents.

The literature informs us that medical interaction is a common site for doctors' third-place sequence-closing actions, performed often minimally, to control the progressivity, direction, and duration of the medical encounter. This chapter shows that patients challenge this institutional norm based on their own volunteered actions and inclination to be effective partners in the process of the meaning-making. Discussed fragments provide examples of varied actions of extended talk as a domain for the limited-English-speaking patient to assert their patienthood. The patients' involvement in this capacity imparts profound positive consequences on the trajectory and quality of their medical interactions. Their post-sequential expansions correct errors of translation, add relevant information, affirm their agendas, and assist the language brokers with the right materials.

Chapter 5

The Distribution of Mediated Text

Who Talks and Who Talks Next?

This chapter is concerned with mapping the distribution of talk through quantifying and qualifying the brokering turn-taking system of medical encounters. In this chapter, I argue that studying the organization of participation in terms of turns' distribution illuminates a critical issue, namely whether institutional norms of interactions add more weight on mutual intelligibility or social membership category as the primary parameter for accomplishing intersubjectivity. If the latter is operationally adopted more than the former, then I hypothesize that patients' voice should have equal opportunities to the interactional floor on the basis of their contextual social membership category as patients, and the opposite would limit patient's access to participation. Three first-time encounters are examined in terms of numerical and descriptive analyses to approximate the interactional zone occupied by patients in comparison to their doctors and language brokers.

Conversing casually is said to be driven by our natural disposition, but interacting in formal spheres is shaped in large by institutional cultures that determine the structure and length of talking. Humanistic is when interlocutors sense that participation and its absence are products of personal tendency or uncoerced contextual elements. The rules of participating may be noted by studying the distribution of talk-in-interaction among participants (Goodwin, 1979; Sacks, 1992; Sacks et al., 1974). Regardless of the setting, processes leading to diminishing context-relevant roles are products of erroneous practices or power asymmetries that interfere in relishing successful communications. In the previous chapters, we saw how our patients deploy various semiotic resources to actively manage their medical visits through and beyond the brokering practice. They proved their agentive character as they fluidly performed their multiple identities to steer the medical encounters in ways that serve their patients' agenda. But how does their participation differ among their interlocutors? How often do they occupy the interactional floor in comparison to their interlocutors? And how often their inputs are accounted as contextually requisite? Through quantitative and qualitative analyses, this chapter is engaged with these questions.

In multiparty interactions, an operative principle in sustaining conversations is the characteristic method of *second order,* which refers to a preference for receiving a response over a selected speaker with no response (Heritage, 1984; Robinson & Stivers, 2006; Stivers, 2005a; Stivers et al., 2009). CA studies have demonstrated that the progressivity of interaction is based on two conditions, a recipient providing an answer and a recipient providing a non-answer, with the latter clearly addressing the relevance of an answer (Clayman, 1993; Heritage, 1984). Generally, it has been observed that "most questions in multiparty interactions select a next speaker to provide the answer" (Robinson & Stivers, 2006, p. 369). In pediatric care, for example, Stivers (2005b) shows that parents refrain from answering questions directed at their children unless interactional problems emerge, such as silence or other difficulties in completing a response. In these cases, the principle of face-saving guides the organization of talking.

Research on mediated medical interactions, on both professional and nonprofessional interpretation, notes the presence of a large number of dyadic exchanges between mediators and doctors (Amato, 2004; Angelelli, 2004). When interpreters perform their duties in the capacity of gatekeepers (Davidson, 1998, 2001), and language brokers act more as caregivers than translators (Bolden, 2012; Del Toro, 2008), the interactional floor could be noticeably narrowed for the heritage speaker. To study how language barriers and institutional norms distribute speakership rights, I examine the frequency of talking in brokered medical encounters via a meta-analysis design. I study patterns of participation to construe the influencing factors as organized by the level of preference to one of the following conditions: (1) an immediacy of conversing on the basis of language intelligibility, thus implicitly empowering the language broker with opportunities to coordinate the information-transferring process, or (2) an adherence to the relevant social membership category so that faithfully securing the interactional floor to carry the patient's voice via or independently from the brokering process.

To carry out this endeavor, I adopt a quantitative analysis to count the number of turns comparatively among participants, followed by a qualitative analysis to examine how brokering and institutional norms parcel patient participation. Discussions and analyses serve the objective of shedding light on the level of attention to accommodating interactional diversity in healthcare communications.

QUANTIFICATION IN CA RESEARCH

The social unspoken rituals of how we manage to participate in conversations and the order of who talks and who talks next are simple, yet fundamental, concerns in CA research, for it underscores cultural norms, power struggles, and the cognitive ability of understanding. In conversation analysis, "the position of the next makes an analytical object" (Sacks, 1991, p. 555) which manifests differently according to the environment. Whereas, in casual conversation, the length, order, and design of the next are locally managed, they are predetermined to a large extent by professional cultures in institutional settings (Antaki, 2011; Clayman, 2001, 2010, 2012; Drew, 1991; Heritage & Drew, 1992, Sacks et al., 1974; Goodwin, 1979). In this chapter, quantifying turns is adopted as a category to measure dominance in dialogues (Markova & Foppa, 1991), it is crucial to acknowledge that asymmetries are irrelevant to note unless they emerge as elements of disempowerment and marginalization. In fact, without a certain level of asymmetry through which interlocutors exchange expertise and experiences, the point of interaction is mute. In that sense, quantifying turns-at-talk is insignificant in and of itself, but the task here is to understand interactional conditions that support or halt patients' speakership.

Schegloff (1993) suggests that adding a quantitative attribution to certain patterns of interaction has always been part of the CA research, albeit informally through quantifying descriptive words such as massively, regularly, or commonly. Increasingly, however, conversation analysts acknowledge and adopt the utility of number-analyses as a robust method to study asymmetries in dialogues in specific environments. However, as Schegloff emphasizes in his seminal piece, *Reflections on Quantification in the Study of Conversation* (1993), even with large amounts of data, the objective of quantification is "studying multiples or aggregates of a single instance" (p. 102). In that vein, quantification should not be understood "as an alternative to a single case analysis, but rather is built on its back" (p. 102).

Three components must be satisfied for quantification to be defensible: a defensible notion of a numerator, a set of occurrences in which presence should be counted as an event and nonoccurrence as an absence, and a named domain or setting for the concerning interactional event (Schegloff, 1993, p. 103). Each of these components requires a well-thought-out determination to avoid casual selection, in which all numerical analyses, including simple counts, percentages, or frequencies, should rest on qualitative case-value judgment. Schegloff exemplifies this by saying that counting laughter per minute to evaluate the sociability of different social groups is interactionally insufficient as people do not laugh per minute. On that account, John Heritage has employed statistical analysis variably in a case study (Boyd & Heritage, 2006), a two-case study (Robinson & Heritage, 2006), and a large data-set study (Heritage & McArthur, 2019). In this chapter, I count the turns of interactional floors in three visits to depict, if sketchily, the equity of participation in brokered medical interactions.

In their groundbreaking work, *Medical Communication in Primary Care Visits*, John Heritage and Douglas W. Maynard (2006), discuss the field development form the initial dependency on statistical analyses to the growing scholarship of micro-analysis. In the introductory review and selected studies of the volume, the authors build an indisputable case for the importance of generating behavioral findings of micro-procedural actions at statistical evidential levels. A number of CA studies have utilized a meta-analysis design of combining qualitative and quantitative methods to reach robust conclusions on social interactional norms (Clayman et al., 2010; Heritage & McArthur, 2019; Heritage & Stivers, 1999; Stivers, 2005, 2010; Stivers et al., 2009). For example, Heritage and McArthur (2019) use numerical and percental analyses to study verbal and nonverbal manners of delivering diagnosis and treatment plans in primary care visits. They note that 35 percent of diagnosis cases are performed without doctors orienting their gaze toward patients and 83 percent of patients who received a no-gaze delivery refrained from commenting on the received news. Through statistical analyses, the study powerfully displays a common transparent ritual of human communication, the preference for being acknowledged through verbal and nonverbal cues when conversing on vital personal matters.

QUANTIFYING MEDIATED DISCOURSE

Wadensjö (2014) notes that normative roles are performed by producing informationally and interactionally close-to-the-original texts, while non-normative roles feature forms of translation that display a wider range of the interpreters' interactive and coordinating actions. The author classifies three types of interpretive texts as reproductions of original texts: renditions, non-renditions, and zero renditions. Rendered texts refer to close interpretations in content and style, nonrenditions are divided into implicit (e.g., repetition after interruptions) and explicit (e.g., meta-comments to coordinate between the two primary partners), and zero rendition are original texts left without translation. Under the rendition term, a few approaches are also distinguished: reduced, extended, substituted, and summarized texts. Most of the named interpretative styles as found in the interpreter dialogue are also present in the examined brokered medical interactions. In this chapter, I adopt Wadensjö's typology to gauge how brokering discourse contributes to the percentage of patients' participation. To understand forms of translation, Claudia V. Angelelli (2004, 2014) conceptualizes medical interpreters as guest speakers of two communities—patients and doctors—but belonging to neither. As such, Angelelli suggests that the interpretive discourse should be examined in terms of text distribution, which could be influenced by adherence to professional principles or an inclination toward patients' advocacy. On that account, this chapter analyzes the distribution of text in brokering encounters based on counting the numbers of turns through which participants hold the interactional floor before the next speaker takes a turn to talk.

Part of the endeavor in this chapter is to draw a rough comparative overview between language brokering and professional interpretation in terms of the amount and direction of translated texts. Amalia Amato (2004) conducts a study on professional interpretation in which she quantifies interactional turns in three professionally interpreted interactions between mothers and doctors at a rehabilitation institute for brain-injured children in Italy. The study shows that the sum of turns produced by the two monolinguals—physicians and mothers—is smaller than the total number of turns taken by the interpreters. Despite professional obligations that advise rendering clients' speech rather faithfully, the author finds interpreters practice a high level of autonomy in judging the content and amount of transferred information. She also finds zero renditions—untranslated turns—to be commonly present in all examined encounters, mostly in the form of patients' requesting help, repetition, or clarification. The author concludes that professional duties are exercised by transferring doctors' talk more than patients' talk.

Through statistical analyses, Amato empirically shows how the adherence to professional identity facilitated by the mutual intelligibility heavily structures the occupancy of the interactional floor. Through a closely deigned study, this chapter examines how institutional and brokering roles affect limited-English-speaking patients' participation

METHOD OF ANALYSIS

The analyses are structured in two sections designed to approximate the proportion of participation in brokered medical encounters. The first section examines three medical visits by means of statistical analysis to quantify participation through (1) counting the number of turns-at-talk per interlocutor, (2) comparing the percentage of turns across the three interlocutors in each visit, (3) comparing the sum of turns of the three interlocutors across the three visits, and finally, (4) counting turns of zero renditions to scale which participants' contributions are transferred less.

The term "interactional turn" is used here to refer to the entire block of holding the interactional floor before transitioning to the next speaker. Through these analyses, this section engages with the following questions: How many turns the limited-English-speaking patients can secure in comparison to their doctors and language brokers? And which interlocutor's turns are translated the most? Accumulated results may sketch a blueprint of interactional asymmetries in brokered medical encounters.

To assess the robustness of the quantitative results, the second section samples the brokering approaches as found in the examined data, selected from three first-time visits chosen specifically to eliminate the impact of familiarity with patients and cases. These visits differ in their purpose and duration, and as such, their similarities and differences may point toward widely-prevalent or generic language-brokering patterns. Admittingly, the small data set may limit the results' generalization, but per Schegloff's argument as discussed earlier, it by no means devalues its conclusion.

Encounter 1: General Description

This visit is the shortest of the three examined meetings, lasting a little over six minutes. Upon entering the room, the doctor immediately directs the interaction toward medicine after opening the visit with a brief greeting and introduction. Three interlocutors are present in the examination room: The patient, the language broker, and the doctor in addition to two observers who remained silent throughout the visit, a small child and the researcher. Nada, a seventeen-year-old high-school student, and her mother, Amal, a thirty-six-year-old working mother with four children, meet with a neurologist to discuss the results of an MRI test. The test was previously administrated at a local hospital upon the recommendation of Amal's primary care doctor to investigate the condition of severe headaches. In this visit, the neurologist reports that Amal's test results show no sign of serious brain problems but reveal a slight abnormality with the nerves around the eye area, suggesting a localized high-pressure problem. To investigate further, the doctor orders a blood test and a specialist visit.

Quantifying the Encounter

The analysis of the encounter shows that the participant with the most turns is the language broker, followed by the doctor, then the patient. Comparatively, it reveals a close approximation between the language broker's turns (41) and the sum of the turns of her interlocutors (45), as shown in table 5.1. The sum of the two monolingual turns does not amount to equal participation, with Amal taking half the number of turns (fifteen) taken by the doctor (thirty); therefore, occupying half of the interactional floor occupied by the

Table 5.1 Amal and Nada's Interaction

Participants	*# of Turns*	*% of Turns*	*Zero Rendition*
Doctor	30	35	0
Nada	41	48	Three of mother's turns Four of doctor's turns
Amal	15	17	0
Total	86		8

doctor. The wide discrepancy in the number of turns suggests that the doctor occupies a fair amount of the interactional floor dyadically with the language broker and reflects the broker's approach in transferring the doctor's opinions. Translation is performed by a summarized-rendition style, in which both the doctor and the language broker hold the interactional floor for an extended period before briefing the patient.

The purpose of this encounter is to relay test results; therefore, missing some common medical-interview phases, such as revealing the medical problem and responding to questions about medical history and examination. As such, the visit's nature limits the space required for the patient to talk since the meeting is conjured to receive the doctor's recommendations.

Zero-Rendition Analysis

There is no occurrence of the doctor avoiding Amal's or Nada's turns. Similarly, Amal and Nada acknowledged most of the doctors' turns with proper responses, but a few patients' turns are received quietly. The patient speaks the least but is translated the most (table 5.1), though three of her turns are left untranslated and unanswered. Contrastively, five of the doctor's turns are left with no translation, because they are treated dyadically or transferred based on summary style rather than verbatim. In this encounter, the turns that are treated without translation or responses are counted as part of zero renditions as long as their transferring carries relevance to the medical issue in concern. However, questions of checking-understanding type are not counted as part of the zero renditions, as they are treated appropriately by the intended speaker, but they make up the total portion of speakers' participation. Every so often, the doctor commends the language broker to transfer the information to the patient, and occasionally, he checks for understanding with the common "Okay?" uttered in a question form. These actions are also left without translation, and they are not included in the sum of zero renditions.

Encounter 2: General Description

The second encounter lasts a little over twenty minutes. The patient, Karim, whom we have met in other chapters, the seventy-three-year-old man with an elbow problem, visits the doctor with his son, Nathan. As a result of a fall, a fluid collected on Karim's elbow, causing some discomfort and worries. The interaction lasts about fourteen minutes and includes all the common medical-interview phases: greeting, introduction, soliciting problem, history taking, examination, diagnosis, treatment, and closing. The meeting ended with the doctor treating Karim's elbow and leaving the nurse to close the wound; the nurse–patient interaction was not recorded.

The son coordinates the interaction by responding to the doctor first then relaying the information to his father. He tries to strike a balance between presenting himself as an informed family member and as a mediator allowing the patient to communicate his medical concerns. His brokering style demonstrates the discrepancy in types of knowledge between an owner and a witness of an experience (Heritage, 2005, 2012; Sacks, 1992). While Nathan mediates as a caregiver, Karim owns the details of his illness account; therefore, he actively occupies the interactional floor as an immediate interlocutor as well as a speaker via the proxy of brokering. Different medical phases afford the two different speaking rights. Questions about the medical history and current medical problem descriptions are usually treated by the language broker as displaying knowledge about the family background, although he often performs confirmation checks. Social rapport and questions about life style or working history are also accomplished by dyadic exchanges between the doctor and broker. Bodily examination type of questions, however, are consistently translated and then answered by the patient. These features of brokering and speakership contribute to the numbers described in table 5.2.

Quantifying the Encounter

The same pattern of turn distribution persists in this visit: the language broker is the participant with the most turns (137), followed by the doctor (104), then the patient (61), but the sum of the doctor's and patient's turns (165) is higher than the language broker's turns (104), suggesting that the language broker practiced some personal judgment over transferring the turns of his monolingual interlocutors. His account suggests that age might factor in shaping the brokering approach and handling the language discordance. In comparison with the previous visit brokered by the teenager, Nathen assumes a higher

Table 5.2 Karim and Nathen's Interaction

Participants	*# of Turns*	*% of Turns*	*Zero Renditions*
Doctor	104	34	
Nathan	137	45	Twelve doctor's turns Five father's turns
Karim	61	20	
Total	302		17

level of responsibility by acting as an informed caregiver. The teenage broker also left some hard linguistic and medical items untranslated, while Nathen treated language difficulties by requesting repetition and clarification. Additionally, varied forms of small talk that register listening, agreement, and confirmation are also left untranslated. These brokering patterns have allocated the number of turns shown in table 5.2.

The Zero-Rendition Turns

As mentioned earlier, zero renditions are original turns that receive no translation. In this study, the turns directed at and treated by the intended speakers are not considered zero renditions. For example, a greeting sequence between the doctor and the language broker is uncounted as part of zero renditions, but it is marked analytically as a form of halting the patient's participation for lasting longer than usual without including the patient. Dyadic turns of confirmation checks are also not included in the sum of zero renditions if they contain zero information that intended to reach the other party. The counted zero renditions are turns that faced comments or no-translation by the language broker, thus they contribute to straining the doctor-patient relationship or the medical information-gathering process. In that vein, I expand the account of zero rendition in this specific context of brokering medical interactions to include some of what Wadensjö identified as a type of non-rendition (utterances designed freely by mediators), if these turns tacitly or implicitly ignored requested contacts between the primary parties.

On these conditions, analyzing zero renditions shows that the patient is the most translated participant. The patient also initiates multiple actions (as analyzed in Chapters 3 and 4) of answering and requesting information autonomously, promoting the language broker to check for understanding through multiple turns. The confirming-understanding turns are left untranslated and uncounted for the zero renditions, as they are a form of exchanges between intended speakers. The seventeen counts of zero renditions are questions addressed to the patient or the doctor, but they are treated directly by the language broker. Similar to Encounter 1, nonresponsive actions to the doctor's questions are not present in this visit, but the wide difference between the doctor's and patient's turns points at Nathen's positioning himself as the primary recipient and respondent of the doctor's inquiries.

Encounter 3: General Description

This encounter reports on the interaction of Salma, the seventy-seven-year-old patient with a hearing-loss condition, and her son, Hamid. The visit is the longest encounter in this project, lasting over thirty minutes and containing all medical phases: greeting, soliciting problem, history taking, examination, diagnosis, treatment decision, a procedure, and a closing. The procedure lasted about four minutes during which the doctor put a molding in the patient's ears to customize her hearing aids. As the mold hardened, the patient became entirely unable to hear such that she was left outside of the interaction; thus, this period is uncounted in the statistical analysis.

Although the patient suffers from a hearing-loss condition, she nevertheless remains active during the visit, excluding the mold-fitting part. Her hearing condition might not be as severe to prevent interaction, possibly also compromised by the close seating arrangement. As she monitors the ongoing interaction, she initiates actions and responds to questions with no apparent problem. Nevertheless, the rate of her interaction is significantly lower in comparison to her interlocutors. What accounts for her number of turns is the son's level of involvement. As an elderly patient, the son's brokering style is another example of assuming a high level of responsibility beyond the interpreting duties. Perhaps influenced by the nature of the medical domain as an otolaryngological visit, the doctor also directs his linguistic and nonlinguistic communication to Hamid, treating him as an immediate interlocutor rather than an interpreter. Although the patient shows a clear attentiveness to the ongoing interaction and responds to all questions, the doctor orients his gaze and talks toward the son while referring to Salma with third-person pronouns. On three occasions, the doctor takes extended turns, which prompts the son to request time for brokering. Despite the visit's length, Salma's turns occupy 15 percent of the encounter, as shown in table 5.3.

Quantifying the Encounter

The same pattern we saw previously persists here, with the language broker producing the most turns (209), followed by the doctor (164), and lastly by the patient (67). The sum of the doctor's turns is significantly higher than the patient's turns, and the sum of all doctor's and patient's turns (231) is higher than the total number of the language broker's turns (209), while the difference between the sum of the patient's and doctor' turns (231) and the language broker's turns (209) is much lower (22) than the zero-rendition turns (41), as shown in table 5.3. Then, the encounter is heavily structured by dyadic exchanges between the doctor and the language broker, as displayed by the wide gap in

Table 5.3 Salma and Hamid's Interaction

Participants	*# of turns*	*Percentage*	*Zero Renditions*
Doctor	164	37	
Hamid	209	48	Thirty doctor's turns Eleven patient's turns
Salma	67	15	
Total	440		41

the allocations of turns. These numbers point to a heavy dependency on mutual intelligibility, rather than the social membership category, which would have secured a fair amount of space for the patient to provide her illness account.

The participants' orientation is displayed numerically by the number of turns and zero renditions. The high number of untranslated doctor's turns reveals that a small portion of the visit is allocated for the patient's participation, while the high number of the doctor's and the language broker's turns suggests that the encounter moves mostly based on exchanges between the two. A unique element in this specific encounter features that two of the patient's turns were translated but they were not answered by the doctor. A few of the patient's turns in which she disfavors the doctor's choice are also left untranslated. In this visit, the portion and structure of the patient's participation are heavily structured by the medical domain and the brokering style of the caregiver.

COMPARING VISITS QUANTITATIVELY

The length and domain of the medical visits can be expected to lead to varied patterns of participation, but the comparative aggregative analysis shows a close percentage of participation across the three visits.

Although each encounter differs a great deal in its purpose, overall structure, and duration, patients' participation differs slightly, as shown in table 5.4. Amal's visit lasts only six minutes; still, her actions amount to 17 percent of the visit's turns, while Salma, the patient with the longest visit, occupies 15 percent of the encounter's interactional floor.

Then patients' participation remains strained by several conditions related to discursive brokering and institutional speech norms. The degree of treating the patient as an immediate speaker—taking in perspective their social membership category as a patient or as a responsibility of the accompanying family interpreter—is a prime condition in structuring participatory patterns. The former affords the patient with a fair space of interaction whether independently or via brokering. while the latter treats the language broker as the immediate interlocutor. This condition is saliently apparent in the doctors' use of personal pronouns when addressing patients with "he, she, her, his," as

Table 5.4 Comparison of Turns across the Three Visits

	Time in Minutes	*Doctor's Turns (Percent)*	*Patient's Turns (Percent)*	*Broker's Turns (Percent)*
Encounter 1	6	30–35	15–17	41–48
Encounter 2	14	104–34	61–20	137–45
Encounter 3	26	164–37	67–15	209–48

Table 5.5 Doctor's and Patient's Zero Renditions

Brokered Medical Encounters	*Doctor's Turns*	*Patient's Turns*
Encounter 1 (Nada and Amal)	5	3
Encounter 2 (Nathan and Karim)	12	5
Encounter 3 (Hamid and Salma)	30	11

opposed to "you, yours, or names." Relatedly, the doctor's orientation toward the consultation time is performed by opening more interactional space for the language broker to respond directly over providing a pace for the patients to give their side of the story.

COMPARING VISITS' ZERO RENDITIONS

Amato (2004) notes that professional interpreters privilege physicians as primary speakers by treating their turns as more relevant to the progressivity and outcomes of medical interactions. In other words, doctors' turns are treated as more pertinent to the medical business, so they are dutifully transferred more frequently than patients' turns. In our study, the patients' turns are translated more than the doctors' turns (Table 5.5). The patients' turns are translated more than the doctors' turns, because a large portion of the doctors' turns are treated dyadically through direct communications with the brokers (Table 5.5).

Qualifying Zero Renditions

Analyzing zero renditions qualitatively reveals varying tendencies in selective brokering. For example, greetings, jokes, and casual comments are left without translation, unless requested by the patients. Turns of confirmation and clarification are almost always treated dyadically by the language broker, whether they are originally doctors' or patients' turns. Patients' zero renditions are mostly initiated actions of requesting or adding information.

In the fragment below, we have seen how Karim takes the time to exchange a dyadic interaction with his son while the doctor prepares for a medical procedure to request a recap of information; the doctor appears inattentive to the untranslated segment as he refrains from checking patients' satisfaction or understanding:

Excerpt (1)

```
282    KAR:  بلكي تنجح هاي.
282a         balki tnjaḥ hāi.
282b         Hopefully this works.
```

283 (0.1)

284 NAT: تنجح،
284a tenjaḥ,
284b It works,

285 KAR: هو يگول ماكو مُشكلة بيها،
285a hwa ygūl makū muškila byha,
285b He says there is nothing wrong with it,

286 NAT: هو يگول وحدة ورى وحدة. يعني إذا مَصارت هاي تصير ذيچ.
286a hwa ygūl waḥda wara waḥda. y'ni 'iḏa maṣart hāi tṣyr ḏyğ.
286b He says one by one. so if this didn't work, that one would.

These turns made the aggregation analysis that represents the amount of talk produced by the patient and the language broker, but they are not part of the sum of talk that reflects the doctor–patient conduct. They are however part of the zero-rendition counts as the requested assurances of the declaration of health come from the language broker, not the doctor. Per the recommendations of WHO, the doctor–patient rapport should include providing explanations and assurances that address patients' fears to insure their commitment to the treatment plan. Interestingly, this recapping behavior appeared in all observed language-brokering events regardless of the LB context or setting. These turns serve to compensate for the limited contact zone between doctors and patients.

Often, untranslated and unacknowledged turns carry important information. Amal's turns in lines 83 and 87 are common examples of zero renditions:

Excerpt (2)

83 AMA: گولي له، يعني مو المُشكلة من المفاصل مال رُگبة مالتي؟=
83a gūlila, ya'ni mū lmuškila min lmafāṣl māl rugba malti?=
83b Tell him, so the problem is not from my neck joints?=

84 =تضرب على راسي.
84a =tuḍrub 'la rāsi.
84b =Pounding in my head.

85 (0.4)

86 NAD: °wait

87 AMA: أني-هاي الاشهر عيوني تغوش, تغوش هواية.
87a āni-hāi aššhur 'yūni tġawš, tġawš hwaya.
87b I-these months my eyes are blurry, very blurry.

```
88         (0.2)

89   AMA: هسة شراح يسوي؟
89a        hasa šrāḥ ysawi?
89b        What is he going to do now?
```

Nada's comment through which she replaced transferring her mother's talk by requesting a waiting period is an explicit non-rendition action (Wadensjö, 2014), perhaps due to language difficulties or to avoid disrupting interactional progressivity. Nonetheless, brokering approaches affect the doctor-patient relationship and the visit's outcome as Amal's hypothesis of her medical conditions are left outside of the gathered data upon which a diagnosis and treatment plans are concluded.

In contrast to Amato's study, language brokers practice their sense of responsibility toward the produced text differently from professional interpreters. Professional interpreters translate most doctor's turns but exercise liberty in judging patients' turns to determine whether they warrant transferring, ignoring, or direct handling. In terms of zero renditions, language brokers demonstrate a reversed attention toward the translated texts. They translate most of their parents' turns but handle a large portion of the doctors' turns directly. On that vein, the underpinning principle of performing interpretation adheres to mutual intelligibility in both brokered and professionally-mediated encounters, but they may differ in the direction of their attention. Both doctors and language brokers are oriented toward a preference of receiving immediate responses, achieved by a shared language. The sense of handling language diversity is also strong among language brokers who, though keen on transferring most patients' contributions, elect to handle many of the doctors' questions directly. The language brokers' common act of responding to the doctors' questions directly is an exercise of caring for a family member, but it also enfolds layers of confidence for handling complicated interactions and displaying a bilingual competence.

QUALIFYING BROKERING APPROACHES

The sequential organization of interpreted discourse is constituted by different patterns and often progresses alternatively from its starting point. All examined encounters are opened by the sequence of doctor's turns, language brokers' turns, and patients' turns, but the order of participation changes as interactions progress, as shown in the excerpt below:

Excerpt (3)

```
03   DOC: okay tell her her ex:am looks f::ine. (0.1) okay?

04   NAD: هو يگول الفحص مالتچ اوكي. مَبي شي. هسّة راح يحچي علامراي.
04a       hwa yqūl lfaḥṣ māltiğ aūki. mābi ši. hasa rāḥ yḥği ʿalamrai.
04b       He says your exam is okay. There's nothing. He'll talk
          about the MRI now.
05   AMA: ah-mm
```

The doctor discusses Amal's MRI results, looking at a file in his hand and summarizing in one-upshot delivery as "looks fine." The language broker reports the doctor's judgment but proceeds to add creatively that "he will talk more now about the MRI," while the mother is attentive to receiving information about her health. This sequence constitutes the default normative pattern of interpretation; albeit, it is not the dominant pattern of interaction as the medical visit moves forward. As the doctor gives his opinion about the problem and its treatment, Nada holds the translation process until the doctor finishes his diagnosis delivery in its entirety; she then summarizes his talk in an extended turn, as shown in the excerpt below:

Excerpt (4)

```
52   NAD ذَيقول المُشكِلة ماما مو براسج، المُشكِلة بعيونج.
52a      dygūl lmuškila mamma mū brāsiğ, lmuškila bʿyūniğ.
52b      He says the problem, mom, is not with your head, in your
         eyes.

53       أه عندج حساسيّة. وذَيشفون عيونج ذَتضرب على
53a      ahh ʿandiğ ḥasāsiya. wdayšufūn ʿyūniğ datuḍrib ʿa::l
53b      Ahh you've allergies. And they see your eyes aff::ecting your

54       الراس، ذَتوجع. يأما راح يحولوج على مـ- مُختص مالعيون،
54a      arrās datūğʿ. yaʾma raḥ yḥawluğ ʿla muxtaṣ māl ʿyun,
54b      The head, is hurting. They'll send you to an eye
         specialist, or

55       حتى يفحص عيونج، وإذا اه مگدر يُعرف شنو السَبب،
55a      ḥata yfḥuṣ ʿyūniğ w̲aʾiḏa ah magidr yuʿruf šinū assabab,
55b      To examine your eyes, and ah if he can't find the reason,

56       راح يحولج على المستشفى حتّى يضربج أبرة حتى
56a      rāḥ yḥuliğ ʿla lmustašfa ḥata yḍrbūğ ʾubrah ḥata
56b      He will send you to the hospital to give you a needle to
```

57 يشو-يقيسون الضغط مالتج حتى يشوفونة عالي لو لا.
57a yshu-yqysūn alḍaġuṭ māltiǧ ḥāta yšūfūna ʿāli lū lā.
57b Se-check your blood pressure to see if it's high or not.

58 الضغط (٠) مال، عيون (٠.١) يگول الخلل مو-
58a lḍaġuṭ (.) māl, °ʿyūn (0.1) yqūl lxalall mū-
58b The pressure (.) of, eyes (0.1) he said the problem is not-

59 يعني، الصوج مو من الراس. عيونج.
59a yaʿni, lṣuǧ mū min arrās. yōniǧ.
59b So, the problem is not with the head. your eyes.

This segment will be analyzed in the next chapter as part of studying brokered medical decisions; for here, it is noted for the brokering style that contributes to the amount of patient's talk and zero renditions. The encounter opens with the default sequence of turn-by-turn translation, and then changes to a summarized-rendition style. The language broker holds the interactional floor extensively and translates by recalling the doctor' speech, causing some information to be lost or transferred wrongly.

Sometimes the holding of the interactional floor is practiced by the physicians, promoting the language broker to request a time for translation, as shown below:

Excerpt (5)

461 DOC: ye-hh-ah so- we'll have you back in three weeks [for-
462 HAM: ahh-m
463 DOC: Ok::ay?=
464 HAM: =let me translate for her

In line 461, the doctor takes an extended turn (not all is shown above), but when the opportunity of a break becomes available by the doctor's question in line 463, Hamid latches his turn to the doctor's turn to request time for transferring the information to this mother.

The brokering styles do indeed affect patients' participation and carry consequences on the reporting content. In the example below, Nathan answers doctor's questions immediately, then confirms the given information with his father. In doing so, he forestalls his father's participation, as shown below:

Excerpt (6)

22	DOC:	so we have (.) pa:in in the right arm,
23	NAT:	Yes sir.
24		عِندك ألم بلـ- بلـ يـ-يسرى، صح؟
24a		ʿindak alam bil-bil- y-ysra, ṣaḥ?
24b		You have pain in the-in the l-left, right?
25	KAR:	لا.
25a		la.
25b		No.
26	NAT:	بابا مو گلت عندك شوية ألم؟
26a		baba mū galt ʿindak šwyya ʾalam?
26b		Dad didn't you say you have some pain?
27	KAR:	شويّة. يعني مو مو فَد شي.
27a		šwayy::a. yaʿni mū mū fad ši.
27b		A litt::le Like not not that much.
28	NAT:	yeah a little not-not that much.
29	DOC:	that is ok,

This fragment displays a back-channeling brokering style. The doctor asks a question; the language broker responds first and then checks for confirmation of his answer. This LB style often finds the circumstance for longer sequences to correct wrong information or add relevant information not provided by the first attempt to answer. If medical time is an issue of institutional concerns, this style definitely contributes to a longer consultation. In line 25, upon receiving the question, the patient denies having pain as the reason for occupying the medical time, which promotes the son to defend the doctor-ability of using the medical time in line 26 (Halkowski, 2006; Heritage & Robinson, 2006) and the patient to qualify his pain in line 27. These sequences of multiple turns are part of the statistical analysis of patient participation, but not part of the doctor–patient relationship or zero renditions.

The *we* is a special term, the kind that puts some burden on the hearing participants (Sacks, 1992). In line 22 above, the 'we' performed by the doctor may represent the formal voice of medicine which endows the doctor with the authority of repeating information that became part of the medical time, such as the patient's information as found on his chart. His use of 'we' in this context may also acknowledge the multiparty conversation and opens the floor for all interlocutors, not specifying if the requested information is a patient's or language broker's domain. The language broker seizes the opportunity and gives an account to an outside-of-his-domain question by reporting on his father's bodily sensation. Hypothetically, if the doctor forms his question with a gaze toward the patient (Heritage & McArthur, 2019) combined with using some form of direct addressee terms (Clayman, 2010), such as "Do *you* have pain," or, "Do you have pain, *Karim*," or even "Does *the patient* have pain," the request for information would perhaps come from the intended recipient.

Below, Nathen's back-channeling brokering style leads to an information-correction sequence:

Excerpt (7)

84	DOC:	okay okay a:nd amm (.) any surg↑eries before?
85	NAT:	y-yeah he got <u>one</u> e::ye surg[ery.(°sadly) yeah
86	DOC:	[one eye surgery,
87	NAT:	عندك-اكو عملية بالعين مو، سويت قبل؟
87a		ʿindak-akū ʿamlyya bil ʿēn mū, sawyt qabl?
87b		You had-there's an eye surgery right, you did before?
88	KAR:	بس بالعين، هيچي.
88a		<u>bes</u> bilʿyn, hyği.
88b		Just in the eye, like that.
89	NAT:	ayy a long °time
90		(0.2)
91	KAR:	لا ليش والله بس مال عين نيثن، عندي هاي مال حصوة.
91a		lā lyš wạlla bes malʿyn Nathan,ʿindi hāi mal ḥaṣ<u>wa.</u>
91b		No oh God why just for the eye Nathen, I have kidney stone one.
92		سويتلها تشتيت.
92a		sawytlha taštyt.
92b		I had the lithotripsy.

In the excerpt above, the son again responds directly to the doctor's question about the patient's medical history. Upon receiving the information, Karim first agrees with his son but then remembers other past surgeries. He uses the cultural discourse marker " والله" /walla/, [by God], which is a religious oath that reflects the influence of Islam on daily discourse (Al-Khawaldeh, 2018), to express his commitment to what proceeding. In this incident, again the back-channeling LB style prolonged the sequence so that the patient may give an accurate account of his medical history.

The micro-analysis of the brokering turn-taking systems shows that the brokering approach indeed affects the distribution of talking. All patients remain active in their way of approaching their healthcare interactions; nonetheless, their participation is heavily influenced by the brokering style by which their interactions are managed. Amal's participation, for example, is limited by the summary type of brokering, while Salma is excluded by a heavy dyadic brokering, and Karim's participation is delayed through his son's back-channeling brokering. Although, all participating patterns may differ in style, they closely approximate in their rate of occupying the interactional floor.

CONCLUSION

In this chapter, we discussed the frequency and features of dyadic and triadic interactions to understand the mobilizing interactional features behind the speaking opportunities in brokered medical encounters. The attentiveness to and the exercise of language abilities appeared to have loud consequences on the brokering interactions and patient participation. Surely, without the language brokers' help, these meetings would be deficiently held, but on many occasions, other's judgments of what materials warrant transferring or not leaves patients defending their right to be informed and included independently, as we saw in the other chapters. In the examined encounters, the language brokers are the speakers with the most turns; they are the coordinators of the information-passing process. This outcome could be expected, as the language broker transfers talks between two monolinguals, but not all their turns are renditions of doctors' and patients' talks. Some of the language brokers' turns are self-initiated conversational rapport with the doctor or the patient, and others are direct management of the parent's health questions. Amato (2004) notes that all interpreters in her study adopt a similar style that leads to a focal orientation on the doctors' talk. This study shows that language brokers approach mediation differently, albeit their orientation toward the doctors' talk is not practiced by translating more doctors' turns, but by answering more doctors' questions directly. Nonetheless, comparative percentage analyses reveal a close approximation across all encounters despite differences in time, reasons, and brokering approaches. The different language-brokering styles operate through delayed, summarized, and back-channeling forms of translation, albeit adherence to the mutual intelligibility in the context of brokered medical interactions is strongly noticeable.

Chapter 6

Brokering Medical Decisions

This chapter puts into full interactional episodes some of the small vignettes we have witnessed thus far in other chapters. It examines the interactional trajectory of culminating into medical decisions from initial deliveries to conclusions. Western medicine increasingly emphasizes patient-centered healthcare by respecting patients' autonomy and recommending shared or informed decision-making processes. This chapter shows how doctors are minimally oriented to such recommendations when their encounters are challenged by linguistic and cultural limitations. Three cases are examined to show how limited-English-speaking patients advocate for themselves to forge an interactional space through which they actively negotiate their agreement, rejection, and doubts about the proposed diagnosis and treatment plan. Initially, doctors appear to follow recommended processes, but they move forward by adhering more to their professional opinions. Additionally, the chapter vividly displays the language brokers' critical position of mediating life concerns versus biomedical concerns.

Involving patients in medical decisions is encouraged by local and international health organizations as an indicator of healthcare quality (World Health Organization, 1978; The Institute of Medicine-IOM, 2003). The rationale behind this advocacy is both ethical and practical. On the one hand, people have the right to their body and health, and on the other hand, their participation cultivates desirable outcomes (Brody, 1980; Emanuel & Emanuel, 1992; Kaplan, 1999; Robinson & Thomson, 2001), such as increased patients' commitment and responsibility toward the treatment plan (Greenfield et al., 1985; Hall et al., 1994; Street, 1991). Despite theoretical and empirical recommendations, delivering medical decisions as a professional biomedical domain that obligates no *selling* is said to be prevalent.

Considering the sensitivity of this context, scholars have proposed different models through which they argue for closing the distance between patients' needs and wants. Two of the main proposed models are *shared decision-making* (SDM) and *informed decision-making* (IDM). The SDM is viewed as an ethical activity in which patients and physicians share all stages of the decision-making process simultaneously, balancing risks and outcomes with patients' values and preferences (Robinson & Thomson, 2001, p. i35). IDM is a legal decision-making process, defined as a practice in which "a reasonable choice is made by a reasonable individual using relevant information about the advantages and disadvantages of all the possible courses of action" (Robinson & Thomson, 2006, p. i35). SDM focuses on giving patients the right of choice, while IDM obligates providers to supply comprehensive information. SDM is most suitable when there is more than one option, while IDM works best when only one option is available. Despite formal recommendations, the practical utility of both models is somewhat vague. Most medical research confirms that decision-making is still practiced as part of the biomedical domain.

Studies reflect an unbalanced state of participation among patients in this medical stage. Richard Street (1991) affirms that patients influence doctors' decisions by offering opinions, disagreeing with decisions, and making explicit recommendations. Contrastively, Christian Heath (1990) notes that patients exhibit extraordinary passivity when receiving decisions of diagnosis, often responding with minimum utterances which can be taken as a green light to carry on with the proposed plan. Some scholars argue that affirming the medical position is contextually necessary. Annsi Peräkylä (2006) argues that eliminating doctors' authority constitutes a context of a nonmedical environment and should not be advocated. John Heritage and Douglas Maynard (2006) note that patients should be invited and encouraged to take part in the decision-making process. Still, the evidence shows that shared and informed decision-making is insufficiently practiced. For example, only 15 percent of cancer patients are given shared-decision opportunities (Meissner et al., 2004). But are patients keen on making their own decisions?

The literature suggests that patients' attitudes might be influenced by different social variables. For example, women, young people, and educated individuals prefer to be involved in their medical decisions, but the largest patient population seems to value receiving information more than making their medical decisions. A study from the United States reports that only 3 percent out of 210 participants prefer to participate in their medical decisions, while 19 percent believe in some form of a shared process, but over half of the survey participants prefer clinicians to make their decisions (Robinson & Thomson, 2006).

THE STRUCTURE OF NEGOTIATING DECISIONS

CA research has contributed to studying diagnosis and treatment decisions in various medical domains (Beach, 1995; Heath, 1992; Heritage, 2005; Hernández-López, 2011; Perkäkylä, 2006; Robinson, 2006; Stivers, 2005) and also to analyzing formats of decision-making (Maynard, 1984; ten Have, 1995; Sacks, 1992). Maynard (1984) defines decision-making as a practice between a speaker exhibiting a position and a recipient displaying an alignment or disalignment with the initial position. According to ten Have (1995), such a process contains three steps: proposal, announcement, and debates, while Sacks (1992) suggests a four-stage process: announcement, response, elaboration, and assessment.

Interactional studies that examine LB decision-making as a standalone phenomenon are limited, especially in the medical context. The infrequent work that touched on decision-making incorporates the topic as part of reflecting on the language brokering practice in general and focuses largely on children's involvement. The early LB work claims that parents submit the authority of making decisions to their children. Lucy Tse, for example, surveyed the experiences of thirty-five high-school language brokers and found that they "influence the content and messages they convey, and ultimately affect the perception and decision of the agents for whom they act" (Tse, 1995, p. 180). Also, McQuillan and Tse (1996) claim that students determine the meaning of oral and written correspondences between schools and parents and take decisions that normally would be made by parents.

A growing line of research has argued that decision-making is a context-specific practice and can be conceptualized as a cooperative effort among participants (Orellana et al., 2003; Katz, 2014). In *Kids in the Middle*, Vikki Katz (2014b) dedicates a chapter to children mediating parents' medical needs in different healthcare contexts. She focuses on the child broker but also includes the perspectives of parents and healthcare providers. Her work shows that the negotiation of meaning-making between children and parents is an organic feature of LB experiences during which parents retain their parental and informational authority

TRAJECTORIES OF BROKERED MEDICAL DECISION

In this chapter, I analyze brokering decision-making in line with two understandings. First, I view the process as a multiparty social interaction constituted by all three interlocutors; and second, I conceptualize the activity as a trajectory of meaning-making with more complicated characters and features than what can be found in the initial delivery-receiving sequence. These two understandings, discussions will be motivated by the following questions:

1- How does the process leading to the final acceptance or rejection develop beyond the initial delivery steps?
2- How does the wide-spread perception of the language broker as a key player in LB decision making manifest when examining an entire episode from the beginning to final steps?
3- Are patients satisfied with participating through the default language brokeree's role or do they influence the process rather independently?
4- Do doctors' behaviors in this phase vary by cases and contexts or do they follow a formally institutionalized mannerism?

Responding to these questions by analyzing full episodes of decision-making in three brokered medical interactions is the concern of this chapter.

Formats of Initial Delivery

Generally, the medical field concurs with respecting patients' autonomy whenever it is safely possible, but studying brokered decision-making reveals a different picture. Physicians usually open the stage by considering patients' right to choose, but they proceed in ways that convey plans designed tightly based on their biomedical views, sometimes even without practicing an obligation to providing necessary details. Within the examined episodes, the following features emerged consistently:

1. The use of the collective *we*.
2. Suggesting the availability of options.
3. Proceeding with a preferred plan and order, which characteristics are not fully clarified at the initial delivery of the medical decisions.

These practices are exemplified in the following excerpts.

Excerpt (1)

235 DOC: th::ere're >couple of things we can do.<

236 NAT: اكو ||شَغلتين نگدر نسويها،
236a akū šaġltęn ngdar ||nsawiyha,
236b There are two things we can do,

237 KAR: ||أي.
237a ||ay.
237b ||yes.

Excerpt (2)

```
211     DOC:     and these're the hearin aids we can pick from.
212     HAM:     uh-mm.
                 ((8 turns of the doctor-language broker
                   exchange are deleted))

220     HAM:     يـگـول إذا حيشدلـكِ سماعة تـخلينـها هِيك ورى أذكـنـي يـعنـي عادي
220a             ygūl āḏa hyšdalki smāʿa txalynha hik wra āḏanki
                 yaʿni ʿādi,
220b             He says if he'll make you a device you wear
                 like behind your ear, like it is ok,

221     SAL:     يـعنـي مَـيصـير-
221a             yaʿni mayṣyr-
221b             So it's not possible-
```

Excerpt (3)

```
20     DOC:    couple of things we can do, I think we need to send
21             her to the e:ye specialist. nd have him take a
               look at her.

22     NAD:    Awkay.
               ((Many turns before the patient's voice is heard
                 in this episode))
```

The above examples show the manner by which participating doctors launch their decisions. The 'we' as used by the doctor provides a strategic double-functions footing (Goffman, 1981). It refers to conversation partners as a group and to the authoritative voice of medicine, and hence a chance to shift between the two. It includes the presence of a third party with a potential to influence the conversation's trajectory and participant's roles.

The second visible feature in the above formats is the employment of lexical items that indicate an action of selection, "a couple of things we can do," in (1) and (3), or "we can pick from," in (2). When more than one option or procedure is available for fixing the problem, the doctors present their treatment plans as an option to be selected from a list of possibilities, as evidenced in the utterance, 'We can.' So, the initial stage of delivering medical decisions is designed following an SDM version, in which doctors invite patients to reach a decision jointly. However, analyzing the developing trajectory of the decision-making phase shows that these options are part of the biomedical realm of knowledge available for the doctors upon which they design their plans.

In this early part of the decision-making process, the language brokers' approaches are partly responsible for structuring inclusive or exclusive forms of patients' participation. In excerpt (1), a prompt translation allows the patient's voice to be heard. In (2) and (3), the patients' responses are delayed and excluded respectively. In (2) the patient' voice is heard after the doctor's dis-preferred treatment plan became clear to the language broker. Anticipating a conflict, the son works to condition his mother's alignment with the doctor's opinion. In line 221, the patient challenges the projected plan with a negative statement verbalized as a question, though left unfinished, as will be explained further. In (3), the patient's voice is not included until much later in the interaction.

Three Case Analyses

Studying the structure of initial decision deliverances may illuminate some aspects of this medical phase as a form of multiparty interaction, but it stops short of providing sufficient knowledge on the state of patients' participation and satisfaction in brokered medical decisions. To further understand the implications of initial decision delivery and the development of the early SDM scenes as found in the examples above, this chapter analyzes the interactional organizations of three brokered decision-making encounters, exemplifying cases of disagreement, agreement, and neutrality.

A Case of Conflict

A concurrence on treatment is a preferred action for doctors and patients, but if dissensus happens, reaching an agreement becomes a tag between two opposite sides. The analyzed visit here constitutes a case of a conflict in which different options are available, albeit the doctor prefers a particular choice and employs various strategies to persuade the patient toward his preferred choice. He even adopts the patient's nonmedical concerns to strengthen his medical concern. As the meeting concludes, the doctor shifts his stance to grant the patient a possibility of choice, at a point in which the patient opts to follow the doctor's recommendation. Thus, selecting the appropriate treatment appears as a trajectory of conflicting agendas between medical and mundane concerns, with a diplomatic third party mitigating in between.

Anticipating a conflict involves employing many strategies to reduce its intensity. In this otolaryngologist clinic, the discrepancy falls between the doctor's preference for behind-the-ear hearing aids—believed to be best suitable for the patient's hearing-loss range, and the patient's preference for inside-the-ear hearing aids—liked for their minimum visibility. This conflict of choices anticipated by the doctor and the language broker. The transcripts below depict this case with their original grammar errors; run-translation appears on unnumbered lines when original turns lay on one-line turn.

Excerpt (4)

208 DOC: Okay, so I went ahead and treated her test results,
209 HAM: Yes-ahh you got here, ohh-okay. ((Pointing at a form))
210 DOC: and these are the hearing aids we can pick from. ((Looking at his computer))

211 HAM: uh-mm,
212 DOC: now this'll show us what hearing aids in that potential
213 range to work for this, hearing loss.
214 HAM: uh-aa
215 (0.2)
216 DOC: nd if we can use (0.1) if we use behind the ear hearing aid
217 we can fit this without any problem. some people don't
218 want (0.1) [behind the ear hearing aids.
219 HAM: [no

220 HAM: يـگـول إذا حـيـشـدلـكِ سـمـاعـة تـخـلـيـنـهـا هِـيـك ورى أذكـنـي يـعـنـي عـادي
220a ygūl āḏ a hyšdalki smāʿa txalynha hik wra āḏ anki yaʿni ʿādi,
220b He says if he'll make you a device you wear like behind your ear, like it is ok,

221 SAL: يـعـنـي مَـيـصـيـر-
221a yaʿny mayṣyr-
221b So it's not possible-

222 HAM: she prefer the small one. ins:ide. >you can't do<, o:r

223 DOC: a sniffing Noise

224 HAM: هسة هو راح يـوريـنـا الأشـكـال الـي الـي الـي، يـعـنـي-
224a hasa howa rāh ywarina laškal li li li, yaʿni-
224b He is going to show us the shapes that that that, like-

225 SAL: هـاي الـورى، الإذان كـلـهـا تـبـيـن
225a hāi lwara, alʾaḏān kulha tbayn
225b that the behind, the entire ear is shown

226 DOC: Well, this is about the smallest one=
227 HAM: =this is a small one,
228 DOC: this is probably the smallest we can get.
229 HAM: ahha

230 DOC: it's gonna look ||like this one here
((Points to a picture on the computer screen))

231 HAM: ||هذي أصغر وَحدة
231a ||hāḏi āṣgar waḥda.
231b ||This is the smallest one.

232 SAL: ayy ((smiling))

233 HAM: تخلينها بنُص الإذان.
233a txalinha bnuṣ l'aḏān.
233b You place in the middle of the ear.

234 DOC: it looks like- this in the ear.
235 HAM: ye:s inside inside the ear, yes.
236 DOC: right.
237 HAM: that that what she prefer, not-not behind the ear
238 DOC: a clearing-throat noise
239 HAM: that what she told me now, ahhh.
240 DOC: is that because she is afraid of what it'll look like?

241 HAM: آه، هاها يگول هاي لأن تخافين تطلعين مَحِلوة، هاها
241a ahh, hahha yūl hāi li'n txāfyn taṭlaʿyn maḥilwa, haha
241b ahh, hahha said is that because you're afraid you
won't look good, hahha

242 SAL: yeah hahah [hahahah hahah
243 HAM: [haha hahahhah .hhh

In line 210, by saying "these are the hearing aids we can pick from," while looking at an image of a graph on his computer, the doctor assumes that his interlocutors are able to follow the logic behind it as well. Then, Hamid meets the doctor's proposal with a "passive recipiency," as represented in his 'ah-mm' (Jefferson, 1981) and no-translation action. As he adjusts his earlier statement to reflect an accurate description of his action, looking at an image showing he is able to understand as displaying a range of possible options to treat her condition. He links the graph on his computer with possible options and assumes that his interlocutors are equally able to convert the science behind the graph into practical knowledge to guide their selection. He, then, reveals a preference and projects a problem simultaneously (lines 216–218). Thus, the initial proposal of treatment is structured through the strategies outlined below:

1- Indicating an action of selection: "these . . . pick *from*," line 210.
2- The options appears to be a computer image of a graph: "*this*'ll show us," line 212.

3- Naming a preferred choice: "if we use behind the ear hearing aid," line 216.
5- Introducing an advantage of one kind: "without *any* problem," line 217.
6- Predicting a possible conflict: "Some people *don't* want," lines 217–218.

In such a complicated manner of delivery, the doctor works on securing his interlocutors' alignment through multiple strategies. He changes his utterances in line 217 from "if we can use," to "if we use," eliminating the contingency of solving the issue from an ability of usage to an agreement on a type. Repairs are locally and interactionally organized actions that operate on fixing a trouble of some sort, and not necessarily to correct what can be perceived as an error (Fox et al., 2013). Through this self-initiated same-turn repair, he performs an action of reduction to fix the trouble source, projecting that the condition for a successful outcome is a matter of reaching a joint agreement. The indexicality of 'we' is yet to be cleared whether referencing the three interlocutors or the medical authority, but he continues to frame a specific choice as the most fitting while admitting its unpopularity. Through a 'no' produced in an overlap, Hamid affirms that it is indeed a nonpreferred option (line 219). Then he translates the doctor's talk showing an early subordination to the medical authority while anticipating his mother's disapproval. In line 220, he mitigates what he understood to be the doctor's decision and tries to secure his mother's agreement. Hamid *sells* the doctor's opinion, using the Iraqi attached future-tense marker "ح" [will], as presenting an action performed soon, a specific device will be ensembled according to the doctor's preference. He ends his turn with a diplomatic tool in "ʿādi," meaning "normal" verbatim, but functionally works as a common discourse marker denoting a similar use as "that is fine," "it's okay," or "no problem." Hamid's turn is a type of an explicit non-rendition comment serves to transfer what Hamid thought to be the intent of the primary party (Wadensjö, 2014).

In line 221, Salma responds to Hamid's actions of selling the doctor's choice with a statement structured as negative, wondering in a question tone about a hypothetical situation, " it is not possible, or is it not doable to," but she abandons her turn, confident that her son understands what she means, as revealed in Hamid's non-rendition action on line 222. Hamid designs his turn in three TCUs: a negative declarative formulated as a question, "you can't," to advocate for this mother's choice, but he abandons this TCU in suspicion of the doctor's alternative inclination, as apparent in the use of the elongated "or" as a token of altering a state of affairs. A question is a face-threatening act (Brown & Levinson, 1978) for both speakers and hearers. It obligates the hearer to give an answer and positions the speaker to accept a possible rejection. Hamid slows his speech as he names his mother's choice but rushes when asking to grant her wish and then ends with a minimum item foreshadowing a problem. The doctor replaces an obligation toward a verbal response with a sniffing noise, which Hamid treats as a rejection, and thus improvises a response, suggesting that the doctor will demonstrate available shapes.

An absence of an action is as significant as the occurrence of an action. It is an undesired and unconventional act, especially in service encounters. Hamid's turn on line 224 intimates the trouble of holding a response when the next relevant action would be nontrivially absent, and the recipient is principally accountable for producing a response. The actions of clearing a throat by the doctor and improvising a turn by the language broker demonstrate how conversation partners are intuitively oriented toward the systematicity of adjacency pairs: if a question is posted, an answer is due as a standard social norm. In line 225, Salma constructs her opinion clearly, saying that the behind-the-ear device makes the entire ear visible, which Hamid leaves untranslated. He transferred her preferred choice earlier but refrains from delivering her dislike here. This visible dilemma of brokering the opposite views unravels the language broker's delicate position when negotiating a sensitive ground. The positions of both primary parties, the doctor and the patient, are clear, while Hamid is in the middle mediating between the two. As his proposal faces rejection, the doctor adapts a different strategy:

```
226     DOC:   Well, this is about the smallest one=
227     HAM:   =this is a small one,
228     DOC:   this is probably the smallest we can get.
229     HAM:   ahha
230     DOC:   it's gonna look ||like this one here
               ((Pointing at a picture on the computer))

231     HAM:                       ||هذي أصغر وَحدة
231a                               ||hāḏi āṣgar waḥda.
231b                               ||This is the smallest one.
232     SAL:   ayy ((smiling))

233     HAM:   تخلينها بنُص الإذان.
233a           txlinha bnuṣ liʾḏān
```

233b You place in the middle of the ear. ((The doctorputs the device in his ear))

234 DOC: it looks like- this in the ear.
235 HAM: ye:s inside inside the ear, yes.
236 DOC: right.
237 HAM: that that what she prefer, not-not behind the ear=
238 DOC: clearing a throat noise
239 HAM: that what she told me now, hhahah
240 DOC: is that because she is afraid of what it'll look like?

241 HAM: آه ،ها ها يـگول هاي لأن تـخافـين َتـطلعين مَحلوة هاها
241a ah. haha ygūl hāi liʾn txāfyn taṭlaʿyn maḥalwa, hhaha
241b Ah. haha he said is that because you're afraid you won't look good, hhaha

242 SAL: yeah. hahah [hahahah hhah
243 HAM: [haha hahahhah .hhh

The fragment above reveals the doctor's new strategy to advocate for a medical choice by demonstrating the devices through computer images. He prefaces his turn with "well" projecting a problem with the upcoming deliberation, in which he describes the device as the smallest in line 226. Hamid downgrades the doctor's assessment to "this is a small one," in line 227, although, we cannot be certain if it is an issue of language proficiency or disaffiliation with the doctor's assessment. In line 228, the doctor also specifies his earlier broad assessment of the smallest available to the smallest 'we can get.' He then shows another picture with the device in a person's ear. Hamid reacts to the image by repeating a positive-confirming token of "yes" and repeating "inside" twice, visibly celebrating the image that represents his mother's preference; Salma agrees. The doctor meets their efforts with "right," in line 236, suggesting reaching a possible agreement, which encourages Hamid to restate his mother's preference (line 237), but now their enthusiastic actions are faced with another holding-a-response action in the form of clearing his throat (line 238).

Hamid uses four persuasive methods to present his mother's case: he declares what she likes and dislikes (line 237), then presents himself as a mere messenger of her words with a laughter (line 239). Through these strategies, he confirms her choice that has stably expressed by multiple actions: a question in line 221, "It is not possible to?" a negative description of the doctor's choice in line 235, a token of agreement, "yeah," and a smile in line 231 when seeing her preferred choice. In 237, Hamid concludes her efforts by detaching himself from her views, which in turn strengthens her position as opposing the doctor's choice. Hamid's laughter in line 239 projects a course of "trouble telling" (Jefferson, 1984). In Goffman's (1981) terms, he animates his mothers' words while positioning her as the author and the principal of the oppositional stance. In doing so, he adds power to her position by saying: "That is what she wants, she just told me." The doctor meets this laborious work with humor as a final strategy to steer this tag-of-choice episode toward his preference (line 240). The doctor suggests that her rejection of the device is due to a life concern rather than a medical concern. Hamid translates his suggestion to a clear statement by altering the doctor's utterances, replacing the doctor's "it" that refers to the device, with a "she", as belongs to Salma, and in doing so he explicitly communicates what he perceives to be the doctor's intent, as saying: "Is that because you're afraid you won't look good?" Salma simply confirms with a laugh.

When the humor does not fruit preferred action, the doctor *fishes* for Salma's agreement differently (Pomerantz, 1980). He now demonstrates both devices physically, starting with the small one. As he puts the device in his ear, Hamid and Salma display a clear preference, as shown below:

Except (5)

```
245   DOC:  okay, this hearing aid [is g]ona be about this si[:ze
246   HAM:                         [yes                      [size,y

247         هذي الحجم ماليتة.
247a        hādi lḥajm malita.
247b        That's its size.

248   DOC:  so it's gonna look about- like this,

            ((The doctor wears the device))

249   HAM:  yes

250   HAM:  شوفي شلون راح تبين,
250a        šufi šlūn rāḥ tbayn,
250b        See how it's gonna look

251   SAL:  أي
251a        ay.
251b        yes.

252   HAM:  راح تبين كلش صغيرة.
252a        rāḥ tbayn kūliš ṣġayra.
252b        It'll look very small.
```

253 SAL: أي أي أي، حلوة.
253a ay ay ay, ḥilwa.
253b Yes yes yes, beautiful.

254 HAM: seem like like-se- it look like there is nothing=
255 DOC: w-w:::e||ll-

256 HAM: =تبين بلكي _|| ماكو ماكو
256a =tbayn balki- ||maū mākū
256b =It looks hopefully-||not there not there=

257 SAL: ||ماكو شي،
257a ||mākū šI
257b ||Nothing there,

258 HAM: yes it look [like nothing
259 DOC: [you can still see it pretty good, right?
260 HAM: yes.

As the doctor demonstrates the small hearing aid as a new method toward achieving his goal, Salma and Hamid go on multiple turns confirming their liking of the small device, assessing its description as pretty and hardly visible. In line 247, Hamid describes the device as "very small," overlapping with the doctor's previous turn. Salma agrees with him and upgrades his assessment to "حلوة" [beautiful], prefaced with three confirming tokens of "yes." Her assessments receive no translation, but the doctor may clearly notice her joyous actions and smiles. In line 254, Hamid communicates their likeness of the device, "It looks like nothing," but the doctor faces their action with delayed and elongated "Well," indicating a problem in aligning with their assessment. His strategies, then, failed to achieve their objective.

At this point, the decision-making process is in a debatable stage, having passed the initial SDM delivery, the first announcement of the doctor's preference, and the fishing for a joined selective action. In lines 256 and 257, Hamid and his mother overlap, almost completing each other's turn, showing an emotional alignment knowing that the demonstrated device is what she wants. Hamid communicates their assessment to the doctor, saying it looks like "there is nothing there." The doctor contradicts Hamid by stating that although it is small, it is still very much visible, then he solicits Hamid's alignment in a tag question, "right?" upon which, Hamid abandons his position in favor of asserting the doctor's assessment, albeit by a minimum token.

Next, the doctor demonstrates the behind-the-ear hearing aids, soliciting their approval through many strategies: (1) re-uttering that it is most suitable, offering more flexibility in dealing with her hearing loss, (2) stating that it does not look as bad as people think, and (3) emphasizing that the visible part outside the ear could be made in grey to match Salma's hair, noting that her hair would cover it. The fragment below shows participants' reactions to this demonstration:

Excerpt (6)

261 HAM: هذي الي تصير بعد-
261a hāḏi li tṣyr ||baʿad ((Gesturing to behind the air))
261b This is the one that sits ||behind-

262 SAL: ||هذي الي- أه-هاي مَحلِوة هاي
||hāḏi ily- ah-hāi maḥilwa hāi
||This is the- ah-this isn't pretty, this

263 DOC: if you <u>use</u> this <u>stu:ff</u> watch-when I put this on,

264 SAL: °لا هاي مَحلِوة.
264a °lā hāi maḥilwa.
264b °No this is not pretty

265 DOC: you only see this and little tube.

((Pointing at the device in his ear))

266 HAM: هذا بس التوب يبين، وإذا ينضم ورى،
266a haḏa bes ltōb, ybayn, wiḏa ynḍam wara,
266b just the tube shows, and if it's tucked behind,

267 DOC: but with her hair you won't even see this.

268 HAM: يگول مثل-اه ها
268a yqūl maṯl-ah hā ((passing his hand on his hair))
268b He says-like ah yeah

269 SAL: زين ليش، ذاك مو زين؟
269a zeen lyš, ḏāka mū zeen?
269b But why, that other one is not good?

270 HAM: which-she asks me, prefer. this one or this one
271 DOC: ha well [I just want to be sure because people when-
272 HAM: [she ask me now

273 DOC: they think about s:ize an the way it's gona look.

274 HAM: ah-uh?
275 DOC: I think these don't look as b:ad specially
276 with people with a lot of hair.

As the doctor wears the hearing aids for demonstration, Salma communicates her disapproval in Arabic, clearly saying that they are not beautiful (lines 262 and 264). Her strong objection is left untranslated, thereby unknown by the doctor; he also does not seek her opinion upon hearing her voice. In line 263, the doctor suggests that the device is not that visible to warrant disapproval, especially when it can be covered by her hair. Hamid transfers the doctor's opinion physically by passing his hand on his head, but Salma remains unpersuaded. She meets their demonstration with a question as to why her choice is not approved. Rather than translating, Hamid elects to present her question as soliciting the doctor's opinion about which device is better. The doctor's answer comes prefaced with the turn-initial *well*, preceded, as normatively does, with another form of a small talk that indicates a change of state or an action of mitigation (Heritage, 2015), uh-haha' in this case, indexing a type of trouble in the upcoming delivery in which the doctor works on repairing his strongly held oppositional stance. As he fails to secure Salma's alignment, the doctor alters his strategy, as in the fragment below:

Excerpt (7)

295 DOC: it is up to her. [either one will work
296 HAM: [Yes yeah but which one is
297 better? That what what she asked me. She asked
298 me about which one is better?
299 DOC: the:re there's really no difference in [terms of-
300 HAM: [the same-
301 DOC: yes, these are different styles,
((Few lines of laughing))
302 DOC: >there' is no better hearing aid< then the one
303 they gonna wear. (0.1) ||hahhahhahhkhaahhah=

304 HAM: ||يگول أنتي- تـ -هاهاها- يگول=
304a ||ygūl anti ta-hahha ygūl-

304b ||He says-I am-hahaha-he says-

305 DOC: =if she's not gonna wear [this, we might as well do the
306 HAM: [yes
307 DOC: other one=
308 HAM: =yes

309 يـگول إذا أنـتِ تـريـديـن ذِيـكَ، تـفضليها بكيفكي. يعني-أنت
309a ygūl ʾiḏa anti tridyn ḏyka, tfaṭaliyha ibkifky-anti

309b He says if you want that one, you prefer it as
you wish. like-it's you

310 SAL: زين، ميخالف دَ-اشوفها. اه-
310a zeen, myxalif da-ašūfha. ah-
310b So it is ok da-I see it. ah-

311 HAM: okay she she want to try which one is better
312 DOC: I think this is better personally.
313 HAM: yes, but she ||want to hear better,

314 SAL: ||هو شيفضل؟
314a ||hwa šyfaḍal?
314b ||What does he prefer?

315 HAM: يـگول هاذي أفضل=
315a ygūl hāḏi āfḍal=
315b He says this is better=

316 SAL: =u:kāy [ukay
317 DOC: [I think this would be better
((Holding the outside-the-eardevice))

Above, the doctor somewhat admits that the patient has the right to choose (lines 303 and 305), but he suggests that such a situation is permitted or preferred only if otherwise she would not commit to the doctor-selected treatment plan. Hamid requests his evaluation and posits that it is his mother's wish, the doctor responds with a faint acknowledgment of the importance of grating her wish, performed with a long laugh (line 302) and an auxiliary (line 305). He declares that if she would not commit to wearing the devise he selected for her, then it *might* be better to stick with the one she selected, adding, with a laugh, that the best device is the one used by the patient.

Notably, the doctor has not yet explained the disadvantages of Salma's preference but dogmatically evaluates his choice as the best suitable for her hearing range. In line 309, Hamid translates the doctor's offer as a solid invitation to give her the right to choose. Salma, however, asks to see them, or possibly try them (line 310), but the doctor treats her request as another attempt to soliciting his opinion; thus, he takes the opportunity to reinforce the superiority of his choice with a strong statement that begins with an evidential verb to express his belief and ends with emphasizing his individuality, "I *think* this is better *personally*," (line 312). Hamid leaves this declaration without translation. Finally, Salma, seeing that her requests are denied repeatedly, she resigns and asks for his opinion, and upon receiving his expected answer, she gives her consent.

The discussed segment of decision-making resembles a tag-of-choice episode that swings effortfully between biomedical and life concerns. The doctor first appears to invite a joint decision-making process to select the best option but quickly withholds his initial SDM offering to support the option he believes to be the best for the patient's condition. Notably, he emphasizes his choice without providing a scientific support against the other option. Throughout the interaction, he champions the suitability of one type accomplished by images, physical demonstrations, images, denying the patient an opportunity to try or hold the devices, not soliciting her opinion, withholding responses, using humor to lessen the veracity of her choice, and equating her choice as only better than not committing to a treatment plan. The patient has challenged the doctor's choice through multiple methods, albeit some actions are left untranslated, while others are strongly transferred. The language broker operates on sensitive grounds as he mediates the two conflicting positions. He carries his mother's voice through, but also leaves some of her strong demands undelivered. Despite the patients' active stance and the language' broker's advocacy, the decision-making episode ultimately tipped to the medical side.

Agreements in Brokered Decisions

Shared decision-making is not always what patients seek. Sometimes, patients are ready to follow the physicians' expert opinions. In this section, I present two cases in which the doctors' decisions are not necessarily met with rejection, but they are accepted actively with questions and doubts. One case exemplifies a patient's agentive agreement practiced through an evidential process built jointly with the doctor, whereas the second case presents a neutral agreement processed through questioning its details. Doctors, as mentioned earlier, deliver their decisions by presenting a few available options but move forward following a solid stance on how each case must be treated. This chapter clearly demonstrates how patients consistently display their stance by treating the presentations of diagnosis and treatment plans evidentially with questions, assessments, and doubts, while language brokers negotiate the ways in which their prepositions may carry the medical and familial voices.

A Case of an Implicit Agreement

In this episode, Karim, the seventy-three-year-old patient with fluid on the elbow, receives his diagnosis and treatment plan. The doctor opens this phase by offering, "a couple of things we can do," then moves forward by presenting these courses not as equally available options, but as a list of steps in which the occurrence of one is contingent on bodily responses. In that vein, these options represent a biomedical domain, rather than a patient's domain:

Excerpt (8)

235 DOC: th:ere're >couple of things we can do.<

236 NAT: أكو ||شغلتين نگدر نسويها.
236a akū šaġltyn ngdar ||nsawiha.
236b There are two things ||we can do.

237 KAR: ||أي.
237a KAR: ||أي.
237b ||yes.

238 DOC: >first thing we can do< i-i:s to try to take fluid.
239 nd take some ov the fluid out, to make it go d:cwn.

240 NAT: اه اه نه- نَسحب السائل هذا، نسحبه ونخ- قَليل.
240a ah ah nh-nsḥab assā'l hāḏ ||nsḥbah, wnx-qalyl.
240b Ah ah nh-we pull this fluid, we pull it out, and we mak-little

241 KAR: ا::ه أي أي.
241a a::h ay ay
241b A::h yes yes

242 NAT: yeah,
243 DOC: nd then we'll wraP the a:rm, so you've to keep it=
244 =wrapped. keep it tied, so the fluid doesn't come back.

245 NAT: نربُط أيدك عَلمود السائِل مَيرجع مَرّة ثانية.
245a wnrbuṭ aydak ʿlamūd assā'il mayrjaʿ mara ṯānya.
245b We warp your arm so the fluid won't come back again.

246 KAR: أي هاي كافي.
246a ayy hāi kāfi.

246b Yes this's enough.

247 DOC: a lot of time the fluid comes back.

248 NAT: وغالباً السائل يرجع (.) مرّة ثانية.=
248a wġāliban assā'l yrja' marra ṯānya.=
248b Usually the fluid comes back again.=

249 KAR: =h:mm.

250 DOC: but that's the first steP, if we can get it to not
251 come back then we're done.

252 NAT: إذا گدرنا منخلي يرجع مرّة ثا- خلصنا من المشكلة.
252a 'iḏa gdarna manxli yrja' mara ṯā-xlṣna min lmuškila
252b If we can stop it from coming agai-we're done with the problem.

253 KAR: خوش.
253a xūš.
253b Good.

254 DOC: if (.) the fluid comes b:ack,

255 NAT: إذا رجع السائل مرّة ثانية،
255a 'iḏa rja' assā'il marra ṯānya,
255b If the fluid comes back again,

256 DOC: then we'll talk about it. (0.1) ||either do-

257 KAR: ||إيرادلها عمليّة
257a ||yradlha 'malyya.
257b ||It'll need a surgery

258 DOC: then we'll do either cortisone injection into the area,
259 area, to keep the inflammation done.
260 NAT: okay what's the cortisone, [g:as?
261 DOC: [it's a steroid medicine,

262 NAT: okay. o::h (.) فـ- فينطيك فد دوة يسموا-مال مالب-
262a okay. o::h (.) fa-faynṭyk fad dawh ysamō-mal mal b-
262b Okay. o::h (.) s- so he'll give you a medicine called for for-b

263 هاي علمود يخلي المنطقة هاي دائما نازلة، هاي-
263a hā 'alamūd yxali lmanṭaqa hāi da'imn nāzla, hāi-
263b This so it keeps the area down always down (.) this-

264 KAR: h::aa

265 NAT: اه اا إذا منجحت العمليّة الأولى،
265a ah aa 'āḏa manjḥat l'malyya l'ūla,
265b ah aa if the first method didn't work,

```
266    DOC:   and if th:at doesn't work then we go in th:ere and
267           we do a surgery to take it out.

268    NAT:   أوكي، وإذا مَنجحت هاي العملية الثالثة، نسوي عملية ونسحبها.
268a          Ok, w'aḏa manejḥat hāi l'malyya lṯālṯa, nsawi 'malya
              wnasḥabha.
268b          ok and if the third one didn't work, we do a
              surgery and pull it out.
```

In the example above, the doctor presents a specific order of possible steps: (1) pull the fluid out and wrap the area, (2) use the medicine if fluids come back, if both fail, (3) surgery is an option. The treatment is presented as a gradual plan with multiple steps in which the utility of each step depends on the healing progress. The presentation of these steps is argued by the conditional particle, 'if;' if this does not work, a next step will be prepared. Karim keenly follows the logic of the plan with small forms of talk, as 'أي' [Yes] in line 287, and 'h:mm' in lines 249, and other similar tokens of agreement he verbalizes upon receiving the translation. In lines 237, 241, 246, and 253, he employs various types of agreement and assessment, such as "أي أي أي" [Yes yes yes], "أي هاي كافي" [Yes this's enough], and "خوش" [Good], demonstrating his attentiveness to receiving the details of his treatment plan. With these various methods of consent and agreement, he also positions himself as a partner in assessing the evidentiality of the treatment (Peräkylä, 2006).

In 257, as Nathen translates the doctor's utterances, Karim overlaps with his son to predict the need for a surgery, an action that is suggested at a later turn by the doctor. Karim's prediction further demonstrates his unwavering attention to the logical development of his proposed treatment plan. The doctor pauses (line 256) upon hearing Karim's voice (line 257) to await translation, and in its absence, he moves forward to give the last option that confirms Karim's prediction; then Karim requires more information:

Excerpt (9)

```
268    KAR:   خوش حچي. هَسة المطلوب شنو؟
268a          xūš ḥağī. hassa lmṭlūb šinū?
268b          That's good (good talk). What is needed now?

269    NAT:   that's good- w-what we gonna do now?
270    DOC:   we take some fluid out.

271    NAT:   نَسحب السائِل هسة.
271a          nsḥab assāl hassa.
271b          We pull the fluid out now.
```

272 (0.1)

273 DOC: okay?
274 NAT: okay.

275 KAR: بَنج يرادلها شي؟
275a banğ yradlha ši?
275b Does it need an anesthetization or something?

276 NAT: are you gonna numb the area? or,
277 DOC: we gonna put some c::ooling solution,

278 NAT: =راح نخلي فد شي مُبرد للمنطقة،
278a rāḥ nxali fad ši mubarid ll-manṭaqa,=
278b We're going to put something cooling on the area,=
279 DOC: =to make the area ahh much less painful.||I mean(..)

280 NAT: ||ميصير بيها-
280a ||myṣyr biha-
280b ||it doesn't get- in-

281 قليل كُلش ألم.
281a qalyl kulš ʾalm.
281b Very little pain.

282 KAR: ها، (٠.١) وهاي تبقى هيجي لو راح يشدها؟
282a hā, (0.1) whāi tbqa hyği lū rāḥ yšdha?
282b Hā, (0.1) and it'll stay like this or he'll wrap it?

283 NAT: يشدها أي مؤقتا (.) وبعدين نشوف شلون النتيجة.
283a yšdha ay mūʾqatan (.) wbʿdẹn nšūf šlūn annatyğa.
283b wraps it yes for now and we see what happens.

We have witnessed small parts of this segment elsewhere to exemplify patients' initiatives. Here, we see the full sequential extension of these actions as Karim fishes for information to build his treatment plan comprehensively. During the silence, he uses the time to confirm his understanding and gives his consent with double tokens of agreement, "أي خوش" [Yes good]. Before leaving the office, Karim also asks if he could use his hand during the recovery period and if he needs another visit (not analyzed here). Karim's contributions show a case of decision-making that goes in accordance with the doctor's plan, while its vital details are revealed based on patient's step-by-step requests. These actions embed Karim as part of the decision-making comprehensive plan.

In this case, the doctor starts with a list of procedures but moves forward with a specific professionally designed path. Notably, those options are listed without presenting any relevant information, such as details on the recovery time and process. The doctor also does not extend an opportunity for the patient to make a decision based on a scientific presentation of advantages and disadvantages of available options as part of informed decision-making processes. He simply lists possible medical solutions, ordered and organized according to his professional judgment. In this case, the doctor does not adhere to his initial SDM nor practiced a sufficient IDM process.

A Case of a Tacit Agreement

This section investigates a patient's visit to a neurologist about a case of severe headaches. After reading the MRI test, the doctor designs a treatment plan that involves ordering a blood test and visit to a specialist. The doctor opens the decision statement in a familiar manner, "couple of things we can do," but uses the evidential verb "I think," to present his plan as a process of seeking for the right course of action:

Excerpt (10)

20 DOC: a couple of things we can do, I think we need to
21 send her to the e:ye specialist. nd h:ave him look at her.
22 NAD: A:wkay
23 DOC: °okay, the other thing that we may have to do i:s ah-send
24 her like to (..)? to get a lumbar puncture. (.) and
25 that's where they put a needle in-you know- like when
26 you have a ba:by they-they do an epidural?=
27 NAD: =Yes.
28 DOC: well it goes a Little bit further, and they measure the
29 pressure to see if it's too high.
30 NAD: o:kay
31 DOC: and if it i:s then we may have to give her pills [(.) to
32 NAD: [okay
33 DOC bring it [down.
34 NAD: [okay
35 DOC: gonna b:e (0.1) a variant (.) beCause everything
36 looks f:ine. and she's getting better.=
37 NAD: =doctor mm she have allergies in her eyes.
38 DOC: she has what?
39 NAD: allergies.
40 DOC: oh °y[eah
41 NAD: [yes [she have
42 DOC: [but this- we're talking about d:eep in the
43 eye.[where y see the ne:rve that goes to the brain?
44 NAD: [oh okay
45 DOC: that's like when I lo-that's what I'm looking at that
46 Pressure neRve. to see if there's any evidence of.
47 I don't see it. but (.) the eye doctor-he puts dr:ops he
48 dilates. can see everything in the eye.
49 NAD: Okay.

In the fragment above, as the brain scans show a healthy organ, the doctor designs a case of a medical investigation consisting of a visit to an eye specialist, a procedure at the hospital, and a blood test (proposed later). Because there is no immediate translation, the patient's response is not part of the diagnosis-delivery sequence. Instead, Nada indexes receiving the information with small items and then asks questions on her mother's behalf. In line 25, the doctor explains the term lumber puncture and exemplifies its usage in line 26 to ensure the language broker's understanding of the medical term. Nada acknowledges his effort by latching her response, 'Oh Okay,' to his turn to index a state of changing from unknowing to knowing (Heritage, 1984). Although the doctor does not address the patient, Amal implements herself as a participant by moving her gaze between her interlocutors to remedy the vacancy of brokering (figure 6.1).

Nada summarizes what she understood from the doctor's speech and transfers information to her mother by an extended-rendition style (Wadensjö, 2014), as shown in Excerpt (11), through which she holds the interactional floor for a considerable long period.

Excerpt (11)

52 NAD ذيقول المُشكِلة ماما مو براسج، المُشكِلة بعيونج.
52a dygūl lmuškila mamma mū brāsiğ, lmuškila bʿyūniğ.
52b He says the problem, mom, is not with your head, in your eyes.

53 أه ه- عندج حساسيَة. وذيشفون عيونج ذتضرب على
53a Ah h- ʿandiğ ḥasāsiya. wdayšufūn ʿyuūniğ datuḍrib ʿa::l
53b Ah h- you've allergies. And they see your eyes affect your

54 الراس، ذتوجع. يأما راح يحولوج على مــ- مُختص مالعيون،
54a arras, datūjʿ. yʾma rāḥ yḥawlūğ ʿla m-muxtaṣ māl ʿyun,
54b Head, it's hurting. Either they'll send you to an eye doctor,

55 حتى يفحص عيونج، وإذا مگدر يعرُف شنو السَبب،
55a ḥata yfḥaṣ ʿyūniğ waʾiḏa magdar yʿruf šinū assabab
55b To check your eyes, and if he can't find the reason,

56 راح يحولج على المستشفى (...) حتى يضُربج أبُرة حتى
56a rāḥ yḥūlğ ʿla lmustašfa (...) ḥata yḍurbğ ʾubra ḥata
56b He'll send u to the hospital (..) so he gives you a shot so

57 يشو-يقيسون الضَغط مالتِج حتى يشوفونة عالي لو لا.
57a yšu-yqysūn alḍaǵṭ māltiğ Hāta yšūfūna ʿāli lū lā.
57b They se-check your blood pressure to see if it's high or not.

58 عيون (٠.١) ° مال-° الضغط so°-يقول الخلَل مو-
58a ʿyūn (0.1) māl-lḍaǵuṭ so°-yqūl lxalall mū-

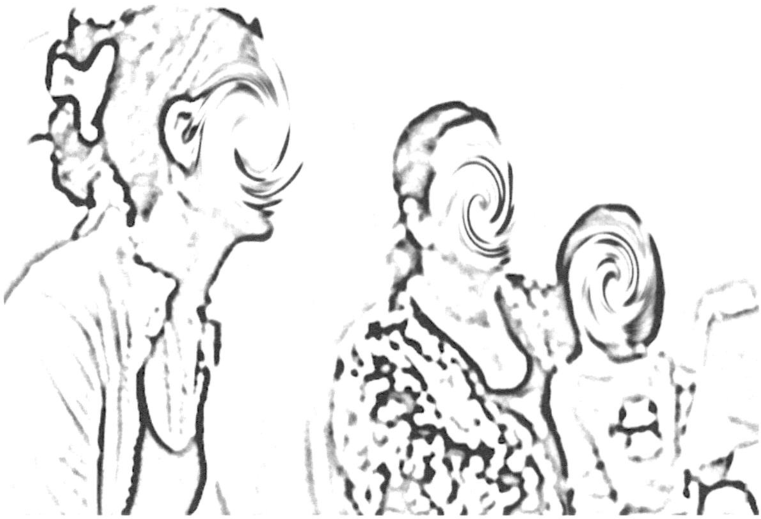

Figure 6.1 Amal Monitoring the Doctor-Broker Exchange. *Source:* Author.

58b eyes (0.1) °of-pressure so-° he says the problem (malfunction) not-

59 يعني، الصوج مو من الراس. عيونج.
59a ya'ni, lṣūǧ mū min arrās. yūniǧ.
59b So, the problem is not with the head. your eyes.

60 AMA: بس گوليلة أني رحت عند أم العيون، گالتلي-
60a bes gūly la āni rḥat 'ind um l'yūn, gālatly
60b But tell him, I went to the eye doctor, she said

61 عندِج حَساسيّة وعندج شويّة بُعد.
61a 'ndiǧ ḥssāsyya w'ndiǧ šwayya bū'd.
61b You have allergies and a slight far-sightedness.

62 NAD: ahh she went to (0.1)||her doctor

63 AMA: ونطتني نظارات||
63a wnṭatni naẓārāt||
63b and she gave me glasses

64 NAD: =l:ike amm <u>eye</u> specialist, and she told her that (.) she
65 have allergies and she ga:ve her glasses.

66 DOC: yeah- but this's something completely different.

Starting in line 52 and ending in line 59, Nada conveys the doctor's decisions, explaining that the main news is that her brain, translated as the head "الراس" /arras/, is healthy. In line 52, she explains that the nerve-irritation case is related to her allergies, a condition unmentioned by the doctor, but Nada relies on her background to replace what she fails to understood from the doctor's talk. The mother informs them that she has recently seen a doctor for this problem (line 60). Although the doctor clarifies that these are separate issues (line 67), Amal remains unaware of his opinion since his turn is left untranslated.

In this case, the patient does not necessarily disagree with the doctor's proposal, but she treats the received information as requiring adjustment. With every suggestion, Amal adds pieces of information that promotes the doctor to fix his plan accordingly. He suggests a visit to an eye specialist, but Amal explains that she has taken that step already; she then requests information about the visit's details: place, time, and cost. Below, the doctor suggests another step; Amal again adds more information as she finds necessary:

Excerpt (12)

78 DOC: and I'm gonna a:sk for some special blood test too, to
79 check [the hormones levels,
80 NAD [okay
81 (0.1)

82 NAD راح يسويلچ اه ه - اختِبار مال دَم (.) ديكِتبه هسّة.
82a rāḥ ysawyliğ ah h-ixtibār māl dam (.) dykitba hasa.
82b He'll order a blood test. He's writing it now.

83 AMA: فحص دَم لو باچر لو عُگبة عندي (١.٠) تحليل هناك.
83a faḥṣ dam, lū bāğr lū ʿugba ʿndi (0.1) taḥlyl hānk.
83b A blood test, I've one (0.1) either tomorrow or after tomorrow there.

((Nada shifts her gaze between her mom and the doctor then looks down.))

84 (0.8)

85 AMA: گولي له، يعني مو الُمشكلة من المفاصل مال زُگبة مالتي؟
85a gūli la, yʿni mū lmuškila min lmafāṣl mālrugba malti?
85b Tell him, so the problem is not from my neck joints?

86 تضرب على راسي.
86a tḍrub ʿla rāsi.
86b Pounding in my head.

87 (0.4)

88 NAD: °wait

89 AMA: أني-هاي الاشهر عيوني تغوش, تغوش هواية.
89a āni-hāi aššhur ʿyūni tġawš, tġawš hwaya.
89b I-these months my eyes are blurry, very blurry.

```
90           (0.2)

91     AMA:  هسّة شراح يسوي؟
91a          hassa šrāḥ ysawi?
91b          What is he going to do now?
```

In line 78, the doctor decides to order blood tests to check Amal's hormone level. Amal informs her daughter that she has an approaching blood-test appointment with her primary-care doctor (by "there," she refers to the clinic that ordered the neurologist's visit). This plan then requires adjustment again; so, the doctor decides to coordinate with the primary-doctor office (untranslated). In line 85, Amal proposes two conditions that could have been accounted for her headaches: her neck joints and her blurry eyes, both remained undelivered. The absence of translation may potentially have contributed to unnecessary tests and a longer recovery period. When turns are not translated, Amal looks for other ways to cast her agency visible.

In the fragment above, Amal produces a number of sequence-initiating actions to understand and manage her treatment plan, demonstrating a meta-awareness in managing her healthcare as well as her family situation. Her question about the place and time of the visit to the eye doctor is transferred by Nada as: "How far is the doctor from here," showing a mutual understanding and management of the family affairs between the mother and the daughter. In this case, the patient follows the doctor's plan without objection, but she adds necessary information with every step which promotes the doctor to adjust his plan.

The above two cases exhibit some similarities and other differences. In both cases, doctors open their decision statements with SDM formats and then proceed with a limited, or hardly any, IDM process. The translation methods have a significant impact on participatory patterns. Whereas the prompt translation provides a space to display agreement and assessment, the delayed translation limits the patient's participation. Nevertheless, in both cases, the patients are actively involved in the information-gathering process. When translation does not come, they ratify their participation through hearing, gazing, and voluntarily adding information.

CONCLUSION

I began my investigation in this chapter with a hypothesis that the medical-decision phase is too complicated of an interactional site to be comprehensively understood from the preliminary way of doctors delivering their decisions. To test this hypothesis, I examined three brokered medical decisions from the delivery phase to the resolving of the encounters. The discussed cases highlight some specific aspects of brokered decision-making encounters, reflecting a highly sensitive mediating ground, where doctors and language brokers oscillate between practicing sharing and autonomous behavior, whereas patients continue to advocate for themselves throughout the entire decision-making phase. Initially, the doctors appear to adhere to SDM by presenting their decisions as a group action, but they shift to a strict biomedical process as the interaction progresses. Perhaps in consideration of the national and international health-organization recommendations, doctors are aware of the professional obligation toward offering some form of SDM and IDM. Nonetheless, they progress with plans mostly built on their professional opinions and show readiness to defend their plans if challenged by patients' or language brokers' doubts.

Interestingly, all presented interactions are not serious life-threatening medical cases, and all have more than one path to recovery. Available options in each case could have been presented with their advantages and disadvantages, allowing the patients to select the best course of action based on an informed decision process. Instead, doctors presented their decisions and plans for treatment commonly formulating their deliverance in a manner similar to, "there are a few things we can do," but continuing by tacitly performing a statement of this sort, "but we will follow this specific path." The information needed to support their biomedical choices are also not thoroughly presented. Instead, most of the important supplementary pieces of information that aid in building a coherent and informed picture about future steps toward recovery were requested by the patients. This phase also reveals the language brokers' critical position, showing how they shift their alignment between supporting their relatives and accepting the medical authority. In some incidents, the language brokers are found to managing the information-transferring process rather freely. Language difficulties, adherence to the medical authority, or a sense of responsibility might be some of the reasons behind the deflation of patients' actions to reach the intended interlocutor, albeit the issue begs future attention. Understanding how decisions are made in the consolidation of patients', doctors', and brokers' actions and studying the developing scenes of decision-making demonstrates the complexity of this site. It is perhaps the most critical part of the brokered encounters where both patients and their language brokers need considerable support.

Conclusion

Final Thoughts

This work cannot be presented in a more timely-relevant sociopolitical climate. In this age of activism of marginalized groups and political climates around people's mobility and displacement, this is the first book-length project dedicated to spotlighting the action and speakership of immigrant patients. Within the feminist movement around childbirth and the work of NGOs in supporting underserved communities, patients have actively succeeded in changing the U.S. healthcare system and professional attitudes, even though no solid definition has been applied to the meaning of their success. In the context of mediated encounters, there are two things to navigate around patients' agency and advocacy. The first issue is to understand what patients want. Do patients want institutionalized interventions to regulate their communications, or would they be more content with managing their healthcare with the freedom of choosing their support system? Do patients prefer to be matched with providers who speak their language, or do they associate providers from the dominant culture with quality care and successful assimilation? These issues might center around the conundrum of giving an illness account, which is closely related to the institutional definition of a patient. In this book, we looked at requests for participation in brokered medical contexts as a ground for studying human agency, sociability, and cognition.

The analyzed episodes are recordings of real-life communications of patients and bilingual brokers from Iraqi families in Southern California with different American healthcare providers. Discussions were guided by a focal interest in the interactional contributions of limited-English-speaking patients when their interactions are facilitated by their family language brokers. Thus far, a profound knowledge has been imparted on the complex nature of speaking on behalf of others, but neither a subsidiary nor less critical is the ground occupied by the person who surrenders to communicate via the proxy of language assistance.

The work has championed the use of recordings in the context of examining interactional competencies of limited-English-speaking patients. Generally, the voice of patients who need interpreting to manage health issues has been absent, perhaps due to the language barrier that conditioned the dependency on interpreters in the first place. Most of what we know about crosslinguistic medical conduct and immigrants' health has been gathered through experimental and reporting research methods, which involve participants and authors with skills in the dominant language. Research that employs real-life vignettes of language-brokering interactions is in its infancy; this is especially the case in the medical context. Beyond a few pioneer works, most of which were reviewed in this book, little is known about immigrant interactions in terms of what contributes to successful or failed medical conducts. Using recordings as a method of collecting data may bypass the language barrier, allowing researchers to witness interactional phenomena as they occur in real time. This is the main argument for employing the method of conversation analysis, which uses recording to analyze real-life interactional events with a foundational principle that no verbal or non-verbal actions are treated prior as insignificant. It is almost impossible to access all details of an interactional setting through reporting from memory, even when assuming that the reporting is objective and reliable. Experimental research also tends to limit the scope of the examined experience and restrict authenticity by generalizing compartmentalized information in controlled environments, while recorded data of authentic interactions provide the possibility of viewing and repeating communications as occurred in real-life settings. Reporting and experimental research methods serve their purpose, but if they are the primary means of collecting information on the state of limited English-speaking patient participation, then we continue to learn about the immigrant medical experience through secondary sources. Conversation analysis offers an operative paradigm based on a foundational belief that social behavior is both context-shaped and context-renewing; and as such, CA analysts approach "their topics by treating the 'real world' as their laboratory" (Heritage, 1989, p. 24). As the real world is steadily and fluidly changing, collected real-life data could continuously serve to reexamine their phenomena against the backdrops of new developments and field advancements.

Through this method, we were able to witness the interactional competence of limited-English-speaking patients operating in contexts intensely structured by discursive forms of limitations and diversity. Interpretation is defined as "a fairly complex form of human information processing involving the reception, storage, transformation, and transmission of verbal information" (Gerver, 1971). The named elements that constitute the process of meaning-making in interpretive events involve exercising individualistic and cooperative behaviors to coordinate interactional progressivity and build mutual understandings (Angelelli, 2014; Wadensjö, 2014, Jansson &

Wadensjö, 2016). In a similar vein, language brokeree's interactional interferences involve mental processes of meaning-making through which they sort out perceived intelligible and unintelligible linguistic and nonlinguistic signs to process, store, recall, and then produce actions to build a space through which they contribute to their medical encounters. They activate these cognitive abilities by carefully monitoring communicational details, even when those details are directly addressed to them. We witnessed our patients responding to complex questions about relevant contextual roles and matters of their illnesses. Karim, for example, confidently responded in English to the doctor's questions regarding qualifying his pain and identifying his contextual role. Despite limited English skills, Karim showcased a competence in English, though limited, but contextually sufficient to constitute a dyadic doctor–patient interaction. Using his heritage language, he initiated actions and responded to actions to specify doses of medicine, anticipate treatment steps, supply his medical procedure with the required information, and participate in assessing the logic of his treatment plan.

Other examples of actuating agentive participation are exhibited by the patient Salma when occupying the interactional floor to provide an accurate and doctorable account of her illness experience. She also challenged the doctor's biomedical preferred choice, demanded to be included in the business/no-business parts of her medical conversations, and assisted her son when informational and linguistic discordances emerged. The significance of these contributions, besides the informational relevance they carry, resides in demonstrating the ways in which limited-English-speaking patients are unlimited by their modest bilingual/bicultural abilities. They strive to take charge of their medical concerns and demand to be treated as active members of their medical meetings.

I routinely witnessed doctors entering the examination room and ushering in the medical encounter by greeting and identifying their patients. However, they proceed mostly by sustaining interactions with the language brokers through direct talking and gazing, while referring to their patients with indirect forms of speech and third-person pronouns. In this manner, doctors opt to manage a large portion of their crosslinguistic mediated encounters by talking about their patients rather than talking to them, as appeared clearly in the quantifying analysis of interactional turns of three medical visits in chapter 5. Those interactions vary in purpose, time, and brokering styles, but they parallel fairly in the active manner by which patients handled their interactions. Despite different internal features across the three examined encounters, participations were parceled into closely matching rates in terms of the number of participants' turns. Although patients consistently work to strike a balance between depending on and overriding the brokering activity to transgress limiting environments, their efforts are often hampered when their actions are met without translation or acknowledgment. Nonetheless, they persist in building actions through which they depart from default expectations, and in doing so, they influence the turn-taking system so that patterns of participation are also altered, as we have seen in chapter 3.

From the institutional perspective, language intelligibility stands as a critical factor of speakership and participating rights, while the social membership category plays a significant role when immigrant families manage their medical visits, as discussed through qualitative and quantitative analyses. Individuals enact their identity as language brokerees and parents by directing their questions and concerns to their doctors via their language brokers. When discontented with the limiting conditions of interacting via the language assistance, they exercise their patient identity independently by using varied semiotic resources to embed themselves in all parts of their medical encounters (chapters 3, 4, and 6).

Expressing the position of informational and linguistic knowing emerges in the medical LB context as a robust interactional resource to assert self-claimed or other-designated responsibilities. It mobilizes not only the sense of entitlement to immediate speakership, but also the sentiment by which a space may be opened or narrowed for others to carry out their own contextual investments and agency. Language brokers exhort serious efforts to coordinate the information-transferring process between their parents and doctors in a dynamic that itself could be facilitated or challenged in accordance with the two primary parties' stances and attitudes. Yet, on many occasions, they enact their role more as primary interlocutors rather than mediators. Their knowledge of the family background boasts them with required materials through which they assert an independent state of speakership, leaving their patients to defend their own speakership and patienthood. This probably explains the earlier claims that suggest the language brokering practice positions. By unpacking the nuances of language brokering interactions, we can see that this sensitive issue is not really about making decisions, as we saw the language brokers carefully advocate for their patients' right and choices, but it is more in the ways in which the interactional sequencing is managed among its participants. This mediated communicational situation persists in this manner not only because of the language brokers' enactment of the caregiver role or their language abilities, but also due to lacking appropriate institutional attention to the complexity of this setting.

This study has hinted at how LB approaches might be influenced by the language brokers' age and language abilities. It was not however a focal analytical objective in this project, because the main purpose centers on how language brokerees manage their interactional contributions despite discursive contextual constraints. Three overall brokering approaches emerged in this project: (1) immediate brokering, (2) delayed brokering, and (3) extended brokering, each of which had different consequences on patterns of participation. Future research may aid in imparting systematic knowledge on how different social variables—such as age, education, or job descriptions of the language brokers—influence interactional mediating skills, and in turn, participating roles.

Additionally, the medical phases also provided different participating patterns. For example, the visit's opening is almost always occupied by a dyadic exchange between language brokers and doctors. Sometimes, doctors close the greeting and introduction sequences quickly to identify their patients direct conversations toward the medical business. On multiple occasions, I witnessed the dyadic exchanges between doctors and language brokers extend to include soliciting the medical-problem and history-taking phases, as in the case of Hamid presenting his mother's hearing problem and Nathen describing his father's elbow injury. Sometimes, patients attempt to secure spaces for their participation by continuing to offer medical conditions and accountable hypotheses throughout their encounters, as in chapters 4 and 6. This interactional norm, in which patients continue to add new symptoms, has also been identified in same-language medical interactions, distinguished by physicians as 'by-the-way complaints;' but it appeared saliently in the examined brokering data, perhaps, due to the limited space available for patients to verbalize their concerns. This is also a considerable element to be studied comparatively in future interactional research between crosslinguistic/same-language medical interactions.

In the medical decision and treatment phase (chapter 6), patients received minimal information due to the doctors' methods of communicating their opinions and the language brokers' mediating approaches, although both elements failed to discourage our patients from advancing their patienthood. Limited-English speaking patients in this study consistently gathered important information about their health conditions and treatment plans, some of what they learned is ought to be included in the doctors' deliverances. Examples of medicate details revealed through patients' questions are: if a medical procedure requires numbing medicine or a follow-up visit, or if the affected area could be used during the recovery period. These types of information are standardly included in preparing medical procedures. Yet, in the cases of Karim's injured elbow and Amal's MRI results, important details were revealed based on patients' inquiries. This element begs a scholarly attention in a comparative manner to impart knowledge on the effect of language barriers on immigrant healthcare.

The diagnosis and treatment-decision phase contains complicated medical terms such as names of diseases, procedures, and medicines. Thus, this medical phase represents the most critical stage of mediating two diverse institutional/familial and dominant/heritage worlds. It is also an emotional stage in which important or serious medical news is delivered. Prior to that, doctors ask questions about patients' conditions, history, and things related to bodily examinations, all of which are materials that could be somewhat familiar to the language broker from previous dealings. The phase of explaining medical problems and revealing diagnostic and treatment decisions involve biomedical forms of speech, some of which could be first-time news. The difficulty of this stage calls for organizing efforts to support the language brokers and patients by, for example, assuring language brokers that the coming speech may contain difficult words and encouraging them to ask for help when needed. Also, doctors need to use gestures to point at body parts concerning medical problems and solutions and to inform language brokers and patients to follow the same course of action when speaking in English or their heritage languages. We witnessed how nonverbal cues operated as interactional resources to help Amal and Salma build relevant actions (examples in chapter 3). Through training and education, nonverbal cues could also serve doctors to ensure the correct information is received and transferred. Patients' verbal and nonverbal behaviors, even those performed with their heritage language, should be noted attentively and interpreted for their value as actions of requesting involvement, satisfaction, or disagreement. In the case of the conflict between the doctor's and patient's choices, we witnessed how the doctor ignored untranslated turns and patient's joyous expressions when seeing the picture of her favorite hearing aid device (chapter 3). Face expressions, body positions, and gestures are powerful paradigms of knowledge that cannot be discounted for the sake of intelligible verbal expressions. Before closing the encounter, doctors should look directly at their patients and ask if they have any further questions or concerns. If responses come from language brokers only, a few seconds of intent pause and gaze toward the patient may contribute to a successful closing of the medical encounter. In all witnessed encounters during my fieldwork, this part was uttered in a hurry (sometimes as doctors have their hands on the door handles) and directed toward the language brokers.

To evaluate the interactional contributions of limited-English-speaking patients, I examined actions in various organizations of the LB turn-taking system, including those located in initial, responsive, and post-sequence expansion positions (chapters 3 and 4). Patients' initiations in Arabic and English represent points of departure from ascribed roles. Their first-position actions are constituted mostly in Arabic through which they ask questions, request summaries, add information, and request to be included in the business/no-business parts of the encounters. These actions constitute the default form of the mediated discourse, mobilized by exercising agency through which they solicit the help of their designated family brokers. These actions also offset extended segments of dyadic doctor–language broker exchanges to build ways for the language brokeree to enter into the conversation via the LB practice. Initiated actions in the responsive position are constituted by patients departing from the default LB pattern to override the brokering process and respond to doctors' questions immediately. They may be verbalized in English (as in the cases of Karim and Selim) or in Arabic as mobilized by monitoring participants' nonverbal cues (as in the case of Salma). An exciting and gripping moment of research was when I saw analytically how the English interaction acted as a nonverbal cue to aid the language brokerees in building contextually relevant actions. With more data, a profound knowledge could be produced to study this element robustly.

When arguing for a sociological theory of information, Harold Garfinkel notes, "[T]he reality of object is not ontological," for an "object has (crucial) constitutive identifies" (Garfinkel, 2008). He argues that an object or a piece of information are ways of approaching the reality of events by placing their faith in a catalog of internalized observations that constitute a broad social paradigm. Garfinkel changed some of his views in later works; nevertheless, this early stance elaborates some universal features of human sociability. Despite contextual diversity, certain features remain as elements of the universal episteme of being in a social structure. By enacting the cognitive faculty of monitoring events or objects, actuating relatedness can be traced to conscious or unconscious agency (Duranti, 2004). To view an empirical exercise of these theoretical observations, the examined mediated context offers an abundant of examples. For incidence, the overall localized sequential structure of medical visits acts as a resourceful object around which opportunities of participation are structured, and as such, provide an effective zone for human agency to activate. Carrying such understanding encourages studying other inherent environmental features and the ways in which they afford participants with opportunities to contribute in limited-dominant interactions.

Previously, the overwhelming focus on the work and psychological well-being of the language broker has contributed to building an unspoken, and rarely contested, belief that depicts the language brokeree as a person communicating mainly in their heritage languages and passively accepting the role of speaking via the proxy of language assistance. On that account, most of the agentive, coordinating, and gatekeeping roles were assigned to the mediator. The examined interactional episodes in this book feature our patients effectively occupying the same roles. They keenly monitor interactions and use nucleus semiotic resources relevant to the structural organization of their interactions. The primary resources that actuate their participation include composing and decomposing prior talk, limited English capacity, and verbal and non-verbal communicational cues. Sometime, they strategically utilize the design of the English utterances as a resource to build entrances into their interaction. Tone, hesitation, repair, laughter, recognizable utterances, embodied actions, and the organic structure of medical visits are example of the resources that afford patients with opportunities to operate on the English exchanges. On these occasions, limited-English speaking patients act as coordinators and restructure the interactional progressivity, while the language brokers and the doctors act more as primary partners. Unconfined by language and cultural limitations, patients embed actions that enable them to sustain levels of involvement whether they are self-selected or other selected next speakers.

These findings encourage medical staff to consider their patient's verbal and nonverbal actions attentively, no matter how small these actions may appear to be. For example, CA research has proved the effective work of small items (e.g., Okay, well, and oh) when used by doctors to control informational flow and interactional progressivity. These studies could be used as examples to demonstrate the effectiveness of micro-actions, and therefore, the necessity of extending this type of attention to understand the actions of language brokers and brokerees.

The adopted analytical frameworks show that the brokered medical text is not a homogeneous discourse, but it has the ingredients of institutional and casual norms. Doctors' discourse in cross-linguistic encounters contains several features similar to those found in same-language medical interactions, such as the use of small talks, including patients' information found on patients' medical charts, structuring consultation time within institutional recommendations, interacting primarily with a mutual language as the primary source of meaning-making even in crosslinguistic encounters, and focusing on biomedical, more than life-concern, information. The language brokers' discourse is structured heavily by their sense of responsibility toward their parents, their levels of bilingual proficiency, and the different medical visits' stages. Despite various contextual challenges, language brokers' speech is carefully designed in ways to perform patient advocacy and diplomatic strategies.

The work also highlights important aspects of the brokered medical decision, one of which is how doctors initially deliver their opinions as a shared process but progress the decision episodes with very limiting shared or informed processes. Examining interactional developments shows that the dissemination of some necessary related information is controlled by doctors, which results in tipping the final decisions to the medical side. In fact, important information about medical procedures and future treatment plans became accessible only through patients' questions. Consistently, patients gather needed information to draw a comprehensive picture of their medical cases, and sometimes their actions lead to adjusting the proposed plan. These findings *silence* claims that allude to patients' passive roles when their interactions are facilitated by their children. The examined decision-making segments are clearly structured by the actions of all involved parties. They are influenced by the brokering strategies, but also by the doctors' strong hold on the biomedical aspect and patients' personal investments.

Consistent with previous scholarship, this study delineates the sensitive and multilayered critical positioning of the language broker. As they facilitate interactions, language brokers often change their stance and framework between interacting, mediating, and translating; thus, actuating multiple roles simultaneously, such as primary interlocutors, interpreters, gatekeepers, caregivers, and information coordinator. All roles have been similarly identified in professional interpretation. In terms of the vitality of brokering, neglecting some of the patients' actions carried some serious consequences, such as unsatisfied visit outcomes and repeated medical visits (Salma), ordering unnecessary tests (Amal), and extending time on checking and correcting information (Karim). More future research is necessary to illuminates features that link brokering styles with mediated medical outcomes. Such scholarly attention can support interventions to build sensitive and equitable healthcare systems.

The physicians in this study managed the medical encounters with some features of SDM but eventually practiced a paternalistic model of medicine in which they controlled the progressivity of the interaction and information. They slightly differed in their manner of orientation toward the brokering practice. One doctor communicated predominantly in the form of dyadic interaction by treating the language broker as an immediate interlocutor, the other two doctors alternated between acknowledging the presence of a group interaction, thus opening occasional interactional opportunities for patients to enter into the conversation, and between interacting exclusively with the language brokers as their primary interactants. Thus, doctors' actions are facilitated primarily by mutual intelligibility more than attention to the contextual social membership category of language brokerees as patients.

While presenting these interactional patterns, this study does not support a specific policy in dealing with language barriers. Despite errors in translation and occasional yielding to the medical authority, language brokers and patients coordinate actions to achieve meaning-making and consider familial situations when making decisions. When planning interventions, the following factors should be considered:

1. The literature shows that professional medical interpreters also commit errors even though they are formally trained to handle medical terms and concepts.
2. Depending on children allows parents to cast control over unintelligible situations; thus, the LB practice may be viewed as exercising authority and agency to challenge the hegemony of dominant social structures.
3. Although their stance my differ depending on the seriousness of the medical setting, doctors who work regularly with immigrant communities

are usually unbothered by the presence of the child broker, believing that they add positive and informative elements to the medical consultation.

4. A strict policy against the use of family language brokers is not the ideal solution. It would not prevent families from continuing to depend on their children, but it will link immigrant communities with breaking rules, which further complicate an already strained relationship with formal institutions. Doctors will also be put in a sensitive position that obligates them to choose between violating rules or advocating for patients' choice.

To build a healthcare system that is responsive, caring, and humane, patient advocacy should be a commitment to establish and nurture from the early years of medical education. Using systematically accumulated knowledge, interventions are must be structured to include patients' voices as critical measure of intervention. Supporting a solid commitment to represent patients' voices, policy makers must build a safe space for diverse perspectives and cultural differences to represent our increasingly diversified society.

Doctors' education must be structured with courses on doctor–patient interactions and crosslinguistic communications by working jointly with departments of anthropology and sociology. To enhance limited-English-speaking patient participation, doctors should be informed about the language-brokering practice in a systematic manner, such as: 1- learning about the ways in which interpreters differ from language brokers in their enactment of multiple roles (e.g., caregivers, gatekeepers, translators), 2- learning about how to provide linguistic and emotional supports to child, teen, and adult language brokers in ways the fit their age and language abilities, 3- keeping a trained eye to spot the difference between triadic and dyadic interactions, and 4- avoid the prevalence of the latter by noting the rates and forms of dyadic interactions and their consequences on medical phases and visits' outcomes. For example, the opening of mediated medical encounters should include a segment in which interlocutors acknowledge their roles and linguistic abilities. Doctor may inform the language brokers on the ways in which patients' voices should be heard throughout the brokering process, while also take the time to acknowledge language brokers' efforts. Doctors can be trained to notice if patients are silent for a long period, if they exhort extra efforts to give their inputs, or if their voices are coming through regularly. A reformed practice must also include educating the medical staff on the importance of attending to nonverbal communication through empirical examples. These forms of knowledge must be delineated through texts, diagrams, and video recordings as instrumental tools of learning.

Limited-English-speaking patients' voice in the healthcare system faces many challenges and that will likely continue after any reformation or sociopolitical changes, but a built-in systematic educational paradigm that enhances patients' impacts on healthcare communication is a potent start.

Appendix 1

The Iraqi Dialect

Table A1 Iraqi Consonants

Arabic Letters	*IPA*	*Symbols*	*Phonological Descriptions*
ء	ʔ	ʾ	Voiced glottal plosive
ب	b	b	Voiced bilabial plosive
ت	t	t	Voiceless alveolar-dental plosive
ث	θ	ṯ	Voiceless dental fricative
ج	tʃ	j	Voiced approximant palatal
چ	dʒ	ĵ	Voiced dento-alveolar affricative
ح	ħ	ḥ	Voiceless pharyngeal/epiglottal fricative
خ	x	x	Voiceless uvular fricative
د	d	d	Voiced alveolar-dental plosive
ذ	ð	ḏ	Voiced dental fricative
ر	r	r	Voiceless trill alveolar
ز	z	z	Voiced dento-alveolar fricative
س	s	s	Voiceless dento-alveolar fricative
ش	ʃ	š	Voiceless palate-alveolar fricative
ص	sˤ	ṣ	Voiced emphatic alveolar fricative
ض	dˤ	ḍ	Voiced dental emphatic fricative
ط	tˤ	ṭ	Voiced dento-alveolar emphatic fricative
ظ	ðˤ	ẓ	Voiceless dento-alveolar empathic fricative
ع	ʕ	ʿ	Voiced pharyngeal fricative
غ	ɣ	ḡ	Voiced uvular fricative
ف	f	f	Voiceless labio-dental fricative
ڤ	v	v	Voiced labio-dental fricative
ق	q	q	Voiced velar plosive
ك	k	k	Voiceless velar plosive
گ	g	g	Voiced stop velar
ل	l	l	Voiceless dent-alveolar lateral
م	m	m	Voiced bilabial nasal
ن	n	n	Voiced dent-alveolar nasal
ه	h	h	Voiceless glottal fricative
و	w	w	Voiced Approximant labial
ي	y	y	Voiced semi-vowel

The Iraqi [r] is pronounced softer than the emphatic trill [r] found in most North African countries. A single "r" is pronounced between trill [r] and flap [r].

Table A2 Iraqi Vowels

Vowels	*Transcription*	*Description*
2 Semivowels		
و	w	High back rounded
ي	y	High front unrounded
3 Short vowels		
َ	a	Low central unrounded
ُ	u	High back rounded
ِ	i	High front unrounded
4 Long vowels		
ا	ā	Low central unrounded
و	ū	High back rounded
و	ō	Mid back rounded
ي	y	High front unrounded
ي	ē	Mid front unrounded

Source: Erwin, 2004.

Appendix 2

The CA Transcribing System

Besides the conventional CA symbols, I created a few tools to work with the Arabic script.

1) = Equal signs come in pairs, one at the end of a line and the second at the start of the next line. They represent latching, a continuous talk of utterances belonging to the same speaker but spread across multiple turns, or they can also represent no break or pause between turns of two different speakers, meaning talks without observing the natural period of transferring talk among conversational participants, such as when a speaker approaches an end of a turn, recognized by grammar (e.g., question) or intonation, (e.g., falling tone), and the next speaker hastes to latch their talk to the preceding turn without a delay.
2) (0.2) The numbers that appear between parentheses in the same turn or between different turns indicate elapsed silence measured in tenths of seconds.
3) (.) A dot in a parenthesis indicates a small micropause of silence, ordinarily less than 0.1 of a second.
4) . , ? Punctuation marks are used to indicate intonation, not for grammatical reasons. A period indicates a final intonation contour, not the end of a sentence; a question sign marks a rising intonation, not a question; and a comma indicates a continuing talk, not a clause boundary.
5) <u>Word</u> An underlined utterance indicates a recognizable emphatic way of talk.
6) (-) The dash shows a cut of speech, sometimes a repeat to repair or to restart an utterance.
7) An *h* represents explosive aspiration, sometimes a small laughter or just a puff of air. In the Arabic script, I use its equivalent sound /ه/.

Hesitation, for example, is indicated with / اه/ [ah], which may appear repetitively as verbalized by a speaker.

8) "words" represents questionable utterances and unclear or understandable talk.
9) (..) An empty parenthesis with dots inside indicates unheard or unclear talk.
10) > < Words in between "greater than" and "less than" signs indicate rushed talk.
11) < > Words in between "less than" and "greater than" indicate a slowed utterances.
12) ↑↓ up and down arrows indicate shaper rises or falls in pitch.
13) ((words)) double parentheses give nonverbal description and extra contextual information.
14) [A left pair of square brackets indicates the beginning of an overlap between speakers.
15)] A right pair of square brackets indicates the end of an overlap between speakers.
16) : Colons indicate a prolongation sound just preceding it, the more colons the longer the utterance is performed. In the Arabic script, I used the colons with the separate letters but used elongated shapes with attached letters, achieved by pressing shift + the letter. For example, ماكو [nothing/not there] is writing in its default printed shape, but مـــاكو is written with a stretched "ma" to represent a longer than usual articulation.
17) For sound lengthening, in the Arabic script, I also used letter lengthening, which could be achieved by shift +J, to indicate the effortful stretching of a sound.
18) || indicates a bilingual overlap. It shows two overlapped Arabic and English utterances, but the utterances themselves do not necessarily appear aligned successively on different lines, as the case with the square brackets that mark overlapped utterances in English. This is mostly to avoid messy layout since the two languages have opposite writing directions, with Arabic starting on the right, and English on the left.
19) Unnumbered translation or transliteration lines are run-on utterances that appear on a one-line turn in the original utterances.

References

Agar, M. (1975). Cognition and events. In M. Sanches & B. G. Blount (Eds.), *Sociocultural dimensions of language use* (pp. 41–56). Academic Press.

Al-Khawaldeh, A. (2018). Uses of the discourse marker wallahi in Jordanian spoken Arabic: A pragma-discourse perspective. *International Journal of Humanities and Social Science*, *8*(6), 114–123.

Amato, A. (2004). The interpreter in multi-party medical encounters. In C. Wadensjö, B. M. E. Dimitrova, & A. Nilsson (Eds.), *The critical link 4* (pp. 27–39). John Benjamins Publishing Company.

Angelelli, C. (2004). *Medical interpreting and cross-cultural communication*. Cambridge University Press.

Angelelli, C. (Ed.). (2014). *The sociological turn in translation and interpreting studies*. John Benjamins Publishing Company.

Antaki, C. (Ed.). (2011). *Applied conversation analysis: Intervention and change in institutional talk*. Springer.

Arab American Institute, (n.d). https://www.aaiusa.org/demographics

Atkinson, P. (1995). *Medical talk and medical work*. Sage.

Atkinson, J. M., & Drew, P. (1979). *Order in court*. Springer.

Austin, J. L. (1975). *How to do things with words*. Oxford University Press.

Baker, D. W., Parker, R. M., Williams, M. V., Coates, W. C., & Pitkin, K. (1996). Use and effectiveness of interpreters in an emergency department. *Jama*, *275*(10), 783–788. https://doi.org/10.1001/jama.1996.03530340047028

Balint, M. (1957). *The doctor, his patient, and the illness*. Pitman.

Beach, W. A (1993). Transitional regularities for 'casual' "Okay" usages. *Journal of Pragmatics, 19*(4), 325–352. https://doi.org/10.1016/0378-2166(93)90092-4

Beach, W. A. (1995). Conversation analysis: "Okay" as a clue for understanding consequentiality. In S. J. Sigman (Ed.), *The consequentiality of communication* (pp. 121–161). Routledge.

Beach, W. A. (2020). Using prosodically marked "Okays" to display epistemic stances and incongruous actions. *Journal of Pragmatics*, *169*, 151–164. https://doi.org/10.1016/j.pragma.2020.08.019

Beach, W. A., Dozier, D. M., Buller, M. K., Gutzmer, K., Fluharty, L., Myers, V. H., & Buller, D. B. (2016). The Conversations About Cancer (CAC) project—Phase II: National findings from viewing when cancer calls . . . and implications for Entertainment–Education (E–E). *Patient Education and Counseling*, *99*(3), 393–399.

Beach, W. A., & Prickett, E. (2017). Laughter, humor, and cancer: Delicate moments and poignant interactional circumstances. *Health Communication*, *32*(7), 791–802. https://doi.org/10.1080/10410236.2016.1172291

Bloom, S. W. (1963). *The doctor and his patient: A sociological interpretation*. Russell Sage Foundation.

Bolden, G. B. (2012). Across languages and cultures: Brokering problems of understanding in conversational repair. *Language in Society, 41*(1), 97–121. https://doi.org/10.1017/S0047404511000923

Brody, D. S. (1980). The patient's role in clinical decision-making. *Annals of Internal Medicine, 93*(5), 718–722. https://doi.org/10.7326/0003-4819-93-5-718

Brody, D. S., Miller, S. M., Lerman, C. E., Smith, D. G., & Caputo, G. C. (1989). Patient perception of involvement in medical care. *Journal of General Internal Medicine, 4*(6), 506–511. https://doi.org/10.1007/BF02599549

Boyd, E., & Heritage, J. (2006). Taking the history: Questioning during comprehensive history-taking. In J. Heritage & D. W. Maynard (Eds.), *Communication in medical care: Interaction between primary care physicians and patients* (pp. 151–184). Cambridge University Press.

Brown, P., & Levinson, S. C. (1987). *Politeness: Some universals in language usage* (Vol. 4). Cambridge University Press.

Brustad, K. E. (2000). *The syntax of spoken Arabic: A comprehensive study of Moroccan, Egyptian, Syrian, Kuwaiti dialects*. Georgetown University Press.

Byrne, P. S., & Long, B. E. L. (1976). *Doctors talking to patients: A study of the verbal behavior of general practitioners consulting in their surgeries*. Her Majesty's Stationery Office.

Cicourel, A. V. (1981). Language and the structure of belief in medical communication. *Studia Linguistica*, *35*(1–2), 71–85. https://doi.org/10.1111/j.1467-9582.1981.tb00702.x

Clark, H. H. (1985). Language use and language users. *Handbook of social psychology: Special fields and applications*. Random House.

Clayman, S. E. (1993). Booing: The anatomy of a disaffiliative response. *American Sociological Review*, 110–130. https://doi.org/10.2307/2096221

Clayman, S. E. (2001). Answers and evasions. *Language in Society*, *30*(3), 403–442. https://doi.org/10.1017/S0047404501003037

Clayman, S. E. (2002). Sequence and Solidarity. In E. J. Lawler & S. R. Thye (Eds.), *Advances in group processes: Group cohesion, trust, and solidarity* (pp. 229–253). Elsevier Science.

Clayman, S. E. (2010). Address terms in the service of other actions: The case of news interview talk. *Discourse & Communication*, *4*(2), 161–183. https://doi.org/10.1177/1750481310364330

Clayman, S. E. (2012). Address terms in the organization of turns at talk: The case of pivotal turn extensions. *Journal of Pragmatics, 44*(13), 1853–1867. https://doi.org/10.1016/j.pragma.2012.08.001

Clayman, S. E., Elliott, M. N., Heritage, J., & Beckett, M. K. (2010). A watershed in White House journalism: Explaining the post-1968 rise of aggressive presidential news. Political Communication, 27(3), 229–247.

Clayman, S. E., & Heritage, J. (2002). Questioning presidents: Journalistic deference and adversarialness in the press conferences of US presidents Eisenhower and Reagan. *Journal of Communication, 52*(4), 749–775. https://doi.org/10.1111/j.1460-2466.2002.tb02572.x

Cohen-Cole, S. A., & Bird, J. (1991). *The medical interview: The three-function approach.* Mosby Year Book.

Cohen, S. A., Moran-Ellis, J., & Smaje, C. (1999). Children as informal interpreters in GP consultations: Pragmatics and ideology. *Sociology of Health & Illness, 21*(2), 163–186. https://doi.org/10.1111/1467-9566.00148

Corona, R., Stevens, L. F., Halfond, R. W., Shaffer, C. M., Reid-Quiñones, K., & Gonzalez, T. (2012). A qualitative analysis of what Latino parents and adolescents think and feel about language brokering. *Journal of Child and Family Studies*, *21*, 788–798. https://doi.org/10.1007/s10826-011-9536-2

Crafter, S., & Iqbal, H. (2020). The contact zone and dialogical positionalities in "non-normative" childhoods: How children who language broker manage conflict. *Review of General Psychology*, *24*(1), 31–42. https://doi.org/10.1177/1089260198963545

Davidson, B. (1998). *Interpreting medical discourse: A study of cross-linguistic communication in the hospital clinic*. Stanford University Press.

Davidson, B. (2000). The interpreter as institutional gatekeeper: The social-linguistic role of interpreters in Spanish-English medical discourse. *Journal of Sociolinguistics, 4*(3), 379–405. https://doi.org/10.1111/1467-9481.00121

Davidson, B. (2001). Questions in cross-linguistic medical encounters: The role of the hospital interpreter. *Anthropological Quarterly, 74*(4), 170–178. http://www.jstor.org/stable/3318379

Davidson, B. (2002). A model for the construction of conversational common ground in interpreted discourse. *Journal of Pragmatics*, *34*(9), 1273–1300. https://doi.org/10.1016/S0378-2166(02)00025-5

de Abreu, G., & O'Dell, L. (2017). Theorizing child language brokering: The example of brokering in health care settings. In R. S. Weisskirch, *Language brokering in immigrant families: Theories and contexts* (pp. 180–204). Routledge.

Del Torto, L. M. (2008). Once a broker, always a broker: Non-professional interpreting as identity accomplishment in multigenerational Italian–English bilingual family interaction. *Multilingual: Journal of Cross-Cultural and Interlanguage Communication, 27*(1–3), 77–97. https://doi.org/10.1515/MULTI.2008.005

DeMent, T., & Buriel, R. (1999). Children as cultural brokers: Recollections of college students. In *SPSSI Conference on Immigrants and Immigration, Toronto, Canada.*

Dorner, L. M., Orellana, M. F., & Jiménez, R. (2008). "It's one of those things that you do to help the family" language brokering and the development of immigrant adolescents. *Journal of Adolescent Research*, *23*(5), 515–543. https://doi.org/10.1177/0743558408317563

Dorner, L. M., Orellana, M. F., & Li-Grining, C. P. (2007). "I helped my mom," and it helped me: Translating the skills of language brokers into improved standardized test scores. *American Journal of Education*, *113*(3), 451–478. https://doi.org/10.1086/512740

Drew, P. (1991). Asymmetries of knowledge in conversational interactions. In I. Marková & L. Foppa (Eds.), *Asymmetries in* dialogue 29 (pp. 21–48). Harvester Wheatsheaf.

Drew, P. (1997): 'Open' class repair initiators in response to sequential sources of troubles in conversation. *Journal of Pragmatics, 28*(1), 69–101. https://doi.org/10.1016/S0378-2166(97)89759-7

Drew, P., & Heritage, J. (1992). Contested evidence in courtroom cross-examination: The case of a trial for rape. *Talk at work: Interaction in institutional settings*.

Drew, P., & Sorjonen, M. (1997). *Institutional dialogue*. Sage.

Du-Babcock, B. (2003). A comparative analysis of individual communication processes in small group behavior between homogeneous and heterogeneous groups. In *Proceedings of the 68th Association of Business Communication Convention*, 1–16.

Duranti, A. (Ed.). (2004). *A companion of linguistic anthropology*. Blackwell Publishing.

Duranti, A., & Goodwin, C. (Eds.). (1992). *Rethinking context: Language as an interactive phenomenon*. Cambridge University Press.

Edwards, D. (2006). Discourse, cognition and social practices: The rich surface of language and social interaction. *Discourse Studies*, *8*(1), 41–49. https://doi.org/10.1177/1461445606059551

Eksner, H. J., & Orellana, M. F. Shifting in the zone: Latina/o child language brokers and the co-construction of knowledge. *Ethos, 40*(2), 196–220. https://doi.org/10.1111/j.1548-1352.2012.01246.x

Emanuel, E. J., & Emanuel, L. L. (1992). Four models of the physician-patient relationship. *Jama*, *267*(16), 2221–2226. https://doi.org/10.1001/jama.1992.03480160079038

Fatahi, N., Mattsson, B., Hasanpoor, J., & Skott, C. (2005). Interpreters' experiences of general practitioner–patient encounters. *Scandinavian Journal of Primary Health care*, *23*(3), 159–163. https://doi.org/10.1080/02813430510018509

Firth, A. (1990). 'Lingua franca' negotiations: Towards an interactional approach. *World English, 9*(3), 269–280. https://doi.org/10.1111/j.1467-971X.1990.tb00265.x

Firth, A., & Wagner, J. (1997). On discourse, communication, & (some) fundamental concepts in SLA research. *The Modern Language Journal, 81*(3), 285–300. https://doi.org/10.1111/j.1540-4781.1997.tb05480.x

Flores, G. (2005). The impact of medical interpreter services on the quality of healthcare: A systematic review. *Medical Care Research and Review*, *62*(3), 255–299. https://doi.org/10.1177/1077558705275416

Flores, G. (2006). Language barriers to health care in the United States. *The New England Journal of Medicine*, *355*(3), 229–231.

Frankel, R. (1990). Talking in interviews: A dispreference for patient-initiated question in physician-patient encounters. In G. Psathas (Ed.), *Interactional Competence* (231–262). University Press of America.

Free, C., Green, J., Bhavnani, V., & Newman, A. (2003). Bilingual young people's experiences of interpreting in primary care: A qualitative study. *British Journal of General Practice*, *53*(492), 530–535.

Fox, B. A., Benjamin, T., & Mazeland, H. (2013). Conversation analysis and repair organization: Overview. In C. A. Chapelle (Ed.), *The encyclopedia of applied linguistics* (pp. 1–3). Blackwell Publishing. https://doi.org/10.1002/9781405198431.wbeal1314

Fuligni, A. J. (1998). Authority, autonomy, and parent–adolescent conflict and cohesion: A study of adolescents from Mexican, Chinese, Filipino, and European backgrounds. *Developmental Psychology*, *34*(4), 782–792. https://doi.org/10.1037/0012-1649.34.4.782

García- Sánchez, I., & Orellana, M. F. (2006). The construction of moral and social identity in immigrant children's narratives-in-translation. *Linguistics and Education*, *17*(3), 209–239. https://doi.org/10.1016/j.linged.2006.07.001

García-Sánchez, I. M. (2010). Shaping practices in translation: How Moroccan immigrant children and families navigate continuity and change. *MediAzioni, 10*, 182–214.

García- Sánchez, I. (2014). *Language and Muslim immigrant childhoods: The politics of belonging*. John Wiley & Sons.

García-Sánchez, I. M., & Orellana, M. F. (2022). Negotiating interculturality from the margins: Translinguistic practices as affective labor in immigrant child language brokering. In M. Fatigante, C. Zucchermaglio, & F Alby (Eds.). *Interculturality in institutions: Symbols, practices and identities* (pp. 295–311). Springer. https://doi.org/10.1007/978-3-031-12626-0_14

Garfinkel, H. (1964). Studies of the routine grounds of everyday activities. *Social Problems*, *11*(3), 225–250. https://doi.org/10.2307/798722

Garfinkel, H. (2008). *Toward a sociological theory of information*. Routledge.

Gerver, D. (1971). Empirical studies of simultaneous interpretation: A review and a model. In R. W. Brislin (Ed.), *Translation: Applications and research* (pp. 165–207). Gardner Press.

Giddens, A. (1984). *Elements of the theory of structuration*. Routledge.

Goffman, E. (1981). *Forms of talk*. University of Pennsylvania Press.

Goodwin, C. (1979). The interactive construction of a sentence in natural conversation. In G. Psathas (Ed.), *Everyday language: Studies in ethnomethodology (pp.* 97–121). Irvington Publishers.

Goodwin, C. (1980). Restarts, pauses, and the achievement of a state of mutual gaze at turn-beginning. *Sociological Inquiry*, *50*(3–4), 272–302.

Goodwin, C. (1995). Co-constructing meaning in conversations with an aphasia man. *Research on Language and Social Interaction*, *28*(3), 233–260. https://doi.org/10.1207/s15327973rlsi2803_4

Goodwin, C. (2004). A competent speaker who can't speak: The social life of aphasia. *Journal of Linguistic Anthropology, 14*(4), 151–170. https://doi.org/10.1525/jlin.2004.14.2.151

Goodwin, C. (2006). Human sociality as mutual orientation in a rich interactive environment: Multimodal utterances and pointing in aphasia. In S. C. Levinson & N. J. Enfield (Eds.), *Roots of human sociality* (pp. 97–125). Routledge. https://doi.org/10.4324/9781003135517-5

Goodwin, C. (2007). Interactive footing. In E. Holt & R. Clift (Eds.), *Reported speech in interaction* (pp. 16–46). Cambridge University Press.

Goodwin, C. (2013). The co-operative, transformative organization of human action and knowledge. *Journal of Pragmatics*, *46*(1), 8–23. https://doi.org/10.1016/j.pragma.2012.09.003

Goodwin, C. (2018). *Co-operative action.* Cambridge University Press.

Goodwin, C., & Goodwin, M. H. (2004). Participation. In A. Duranti (Ed.), *Companion to linguistic anthropology* (pp. 222–244). Blackwell Publishing. https://doi.org/10.1002/9780470996522

Goodwin, C., & Heritage, J. (1990). Conversation analysis. *Annual Review of Anthropology*, *19*(1), 283–307. https://doi.org/10.1146/annurev.an.19.100190.001435

Goodwin, M. H., & Goodwin, C. (1986). Gesture and co-participation in the activity of searching for a word. https://doi.org/10.1515/semi.1986.62.1-2.51

Goodwin, M. H. (1990). *He-said-she-said: Talk as social organization among black children.* Indiana University Press.

Greenfield, S., Kaplan, S., & Ware Jr, J. (1985). Expanding patient involvement in care: Effects on patient outcomes. *Annals of Internal Medicine*, *102*(4), 520–528. https://doi.org/10.7326/0003-4819-102-4-520

Guan, S. S. A., Nash, A., & Orellana, M. F. (2016). Cultural and social processes of language brokering among Arab, Asian, and Latin immigrants. *Journal of Multilingual and Multicultural Development*, *37*(2), 150–166. https://doi.org/10.1080/01434632.2015.1044997

Gumperz, J. J. (1981). Conversational inference and classroom learning. In J. Green & C. Wallat (Eds.), *Ethnography and language in educational settings* (pp. 2–23). Ablex.

Hadziabdic, E., & Hjelm, K. (2014). Arabic-speaking migrants' experiences of the use of interpreters in healthcare: A qualitative explorative study. *International Journal for Equity in Health*, *13*(49), 1–12. https://doi.org/10.1186/1475-9276-13-49

Halkowski, T. (2006). Realizing the illness: Patients' narratives of symptom discovery. In J. Heritage & D. W. Maynard (Eds.), *Communication in medical care: Interaction between primary care physicians and patient* (pp. 151–184). Cambridge University Press.

Hall, J. A., Irish, J. T., Roter, D. L., Ehrlich, M. C., & Miller, L. H. (1994). Satisfaction, gender, and communication in medical visits. *Medical Care*, 1216–1231. https://www.jstor.org/stable/3766526

Hall, N., & Robinson, A. (1999). The language brokering behaviour of young children in families of Pakistani heritage. *Unpublished research report.*

Harris, B. (1973). *The importance of natural translation.* University of Ottawa.

Heath, C. (1986). *Body movement and speech in medical interaction*. Cambridge University Press.

Heath, C. (1992). The delivery and reception of diagnosis in the general-practice consultations. In P. Drew & J. Heritage (Eds.), *Talk at work: Studies in interactional sociolinguistics* (pp. 235–267). Cambridge University Press.

Hepburn, A., & Bolden, G. B. (2012). The conversation analysis approach to transcription. In T. Stivers & J. Sidnell (Eds.), *The handbook of conversation analysis* (57–76). Blackwell.

Heritage, J. (1984). A change-of-state token and aspects of its sequential placement. *Structures of Social Action: Studies in Conversation Analysis*, 299–345.

Heritage, J. (1988). Explanations as accounts: A conversation analytic perspective. In C. Antaki (Ed.), *Analysing everyday explanation: A casebook of methods* (pp. 127–144). Sage Publications, Inc.

Heritage, J. (1989). Current developments in conversation analysis. In D. Roger & P. Bull (Eds.), *Conversation: An interdisciplinary perspective* (pp. 21–47). Multilingual Matters.

Heritage, J. (2002). The limits of questioning: Negative interrogatives and hostile question content. *Journal of Pragmatics*, *34*(10–11), 1427–1446. https://doi.org/10.1016/S0378-2166(02)00072-3

Heritage, J. (2005). Conversation analysis and institutional talk. In K. L. Fitch & R. E. Sanders (Eds.), *Handbook of language and social interaction* (pp. 103–147). Psychology Press.

Heritage, J. (2008). Conversation analysis as social theory. In B. S. Turner (Ed.), *The new Blackwell companion to social theory* (pp. 300–320). Wiley Blackwell.

Heritage, J. (2010). Questioning in medicine. In A. F. Freed & S. Ehrlich (Eds.), *Why do you ask: The function of questions in institutional discourse* (pp. 42–68). Oxford University Press.

Heritage, J. (2012). Epistemics in action: Action formation and territories of knowledge. *Research on Language & Social Interaction*, *45*(1).1–29. https://doi.org/10.1080/08351813.2012.646684

Heritage, J. (2015). Well-prefaced turns in English conversation: A conversation analytic perspective. *Journal of Pragmatics*, *88*, 88–104.

Heritage, J., & Clayman, S. (2011). *Talk in action: Interactions, identities, and institutions*. Wiley-Blackwell.

Heritage, J., & Drew, P. (1992). Talk at work. *Interaction in institutional settings*. Cambridge University Press.

Heritage, J., & McArthur, A. (2019). The diagnostic moment: A study in US primary care. *Social Science & Medicine*, *228*, 262–271. https://doi.org/10.1016/j.socscimed.2019.03.022

Heritage, J., Robinson, J. D., Elliott, M. N., Beckett, M., & Wilkes, M. (2007). Reducing patients' unmet concerns in primary care: The difference one word can make. *Journal of General Internal Medicine*, *22*, 1429–1433. https://doi.org/10.1007/s11606-007-0279-0

Heritage, J.& Raymond, G. (2005). The terms of agreement: Indexing epistemic authority and subordination in talk-in-interaction. *Social Psychology Quarterly*, *68*(1), 15–38. https://doi.org/10.1177/019027250506800103

Heritage, J., & Robinson, J. D. (2006). Accounting for the visit: Giving reasons for seeking medical care. *Studies in Interactional Sociolinguistics 20*, 48.

Heritage, J., & Sefi, S. (1992) Dilemmas of advice: Aspects of the delivery and reception of advice in interactions between health visitors and first-time mothers. In P. Drew & J. Heritage (Eds.), *Talk at work: Interaction in institutional settings* (359, 417). Cambridge University Press.

Heritage, J., & Stivers, T. (1999). Online commentary in acute medical visits: A method of shaping patient expectations. *Social Science & Medicine*, *49*(11), 1501–1517. https://doi.org/10.1016/S0277-9536(99)00219-1

Hoffman, B., Tomes, N., Grob, R., & Schlesinger, M. (Eds.). (2011). *Patients as policy actors: A century of changing markets and missions*. Rutgers University Press.

Holmes-Eber, P. (2020). Redefining the past to become the present: Culture policy and US marine corps recruit training. In K. Enstad & P. Holmes-Eber (Eds.), *Warriors or peacekeepers? Building military cultural competence* (pp. 205–224). Springer.

Hua, J. M., & Costigan, C. L. (2017). Adolescent language brokering for immigrant Chinese parents in Canada. In R. S. Weisskirch (Ed.), *Language brokering in immigrant families: Theories and contexts* (pp. 137–159). Routledge.

Hymez, D. H. (1974). *Foundations in sociolinguistics: An ethnography approach*. University of Pennsylvania Press.

Institute of Medicine US, Committee on Assuring the Health of the Public in the 21st Century, Committee on Assuring the Health of the Public in the 21st Century, Institute of Medicine, Board on Health Promotion, & Disease Prevention. (2003). *The future of the public's health in the 21st century*. National Academy Press.

Jacknick, C. M. (2011). "But this is writing": Post-expansion in student-initiated sequences. *Novitas-ROYAL* (Research on Youth and Language), *5*(1), 39–54

Jacoby, S., & Ochs, E. (1995). Co-construction: An introduction. *Research on Language and Social Interaction*, *29*(3), 171–183. https://doi.org/10.1207/s15327973rlsi28031

Jansson, G., & Wadensjö, C. (2016). Language brokering in multilingual caregiving settings. *Communication and Medicine: An interdisciplinary Journal of Healthcare, Ethics, and Society*, 13(3), 277–290.

Jefferson, G., & Lee, J. R. (1981). The rejection of advice: Managing the problematic convergence of a 'troubles-telling' and a 'service encounter.' *Journal of Pragmatics*, *5*(5), 399–422. https://doi.org/10.1016/0378-2166(81)90026-6

Jones, C. J., & Trickett, E. J. (2005). Immigrant adolescents behaving as culture brokers: A study of families from the former Soviet Union. *The Journal of Social Psychology*, *145*(4), 405–428. https://doi.org/10.3200/SOCP. 145.4.405-428

Kaplan, R. M. (1999). Shared medical decision-making: A new paradigm for behavioral medicine—1997 presidential address. *Annals of Behavioral Medicine*, *21*(1), 3–11. https://doi.org/10.1007/BF02895027

Katz, V. S. (2014a). Children as brokers of their immigrant families' health-care connections. *Social Problems*, *61*(2), 194–215. https://doi.org/10.1525/sp. 2014.12026

Katz, V. S. (2014b). *Kids in the middle: How children of immigrants negotiate community interactions for their families*. Rutgers University Press.

Kaufert, J. M., & Putsch, R. W. (1997). Communication through interpreters in healthcare: Ethical dilemmas arising from differences in class, culture, language, and power. *The Journal of Clinical Ethics*, *8*(1), 71–87.

Kim, S. Y., Zhang, M., Chen, S., Song, J., Lopez, B. G., Rodriguez, E. M., & Shen, Y. (2020). Bilingual language broker profiles and academic competence in Mexican-origin adolescents. *Developmental Psychology*, *56*(8), 1582.

Lee, K. C., Winickoff, J. P., Kim, M. K., Campbell, E. G., Betancourt, J. R., Park, E. R., & Weissman, J. S. (2006). Resident physicians' use of professional and nonprofessional interpreters: A national survey. *Jama*, *296*(9), 1049–1105. https://doi.org/10.1001/jama.296.9.1050

Lee, N., Mikesell, L., Joaquin, A. D. L., Mates, A. W., & Schumann, J. H. (2009). *The interactional instinct: The evolution and acquisition of language*. Oxford University Press.

Love, J. A., & Buriel, R. (2007). Language brokering, autonomy, parent-child bonding, biculturalism, and depression: A study of Mexican American adolescents from immigrant families. *Hispanic Journal of Behavioral Sciences*, *29*(4), 472–491. https://doi.org/10.1177/0739986307307229

Markova, I., & Foppa, K. (1991). *Asymmetries in dialogue 29*. Harvester Wheatsheaf.

Malakoff, M., & Hakuta, K. (1991). Translation skill and metalinguistic awareness in bilinguals. In E. Bialystock (Ed.), *Language processing in bilingual children* (pp. 141–166). Cambridge University Press.

Martinez, K., Orellana, M. F., Murillo, M. A., & Rodriguez, M. A. (2017). Health insurance, from a child language broker's perspective. *International Migration*, *55*(5), 31–43. https://doi.org/10.1111/imig.12380

Maynard, D. W. (1984). *Inside plea bargaining*. Springer. https://doi.org/10.1207/s15327973rlsi3002_1

Maynard, D. W. (1997). The news delivery sequence: Bad news and good news in conversational interaction. *Research on Language and Social Interaction*, *30*(2), 93–130.

Maynard, D. W., & Heritage, J. (2005). Conversation analysis, doctor–patient interaction and medical communication. *Medical Education*, *39*(4), 428–435. https://doi.org/10.1111/j.1365-2929.2005.02111.x

McQuillan, J., & Tse, L (1995). Child language brokering in linguistic minority communities: effects on cultural interaction, cognition, and literacy. *Language and Education*, *9*(3), 195–215. https://doi.org/10.1080/09500789509541413

Meissner, H. I., Smith, R. A., Rimer, B. K., Wilson, K. M., Rakowski, W., Vernon, S. W., & Briss, P. A. (2004). Promoting cancer screening: Learning from experience. *Cancer: Interdisciplinary International Journal of the American Cancer Society*, *101*(S5), 1107–1117. https://doi.org/10.1002/cncr.20507

Mishler, E. G. (1984). *The discourse of medicine: Dialectics of medical interviews* (Vol. 3). Greenwood Publishing Group.

Nash, A. (2017). Arab Americans brokering in a context of tension and stereotypes: "It's just a head-cover. get over it!." In R. S. Weisskirch (Ed.), *Language brokering in immigrant families: Theories and contexts* (pp. 116–136). Routledge.

Nash, A. (2022). Arabic in greater Los Angeles: Many varieties, one community. In Chik, C. H. (Ed.), *Multilingual La La Land: Language use in sixteen Greater Los Angeles communities* (pp. 7–27). Routledge.

Ochs, E., & Schieffelin, B. B. (2016). *Acquiring conversational competence*. Routledge.

Ochs, E., & Solomon, O. (2010). Autistic sociality. *Ethos*, *38*(1), 69–92. https://doi.org/10.1111/j.1548-1352.2009.01082.x

Orellana, M. F. (2001). The work kids do: Mexican and Central American immigrant children's contributions to households and schools in California. *Harvard Educational Review*, *71*(3), 366–390. https://doi.org/10.17763/haer.71.3.52320g7n21922hw4

Orellana, M. F. (2003). Responsibilities of children in Latino immigrant homes. *New directions for youth development*, *2003*(100), 25–39. https://doi.org/10.1002/yd.61

Orellana, M. F. (2009). *Translating childhoods: Immigrant youth, language, and culture*. Rutgers University Press.

Orellana, M. F. (2015). *Immigrant children in transcultural spaces: Language, learning, and love*. Routledge.

Orellana, M. F., Dorner, L., & Pulido, L. (2008). Accessing assets: Immigrant youth's work as family translators or "para-phrasers." *Social Problems*, *50*(4), 505–524. nhttps://doi.org/10.1525/sp. 2003.50.4.505

Orellana, M. F., Martínez, D. C., Lee, C. H., & Montaño, E. (2012). Language as a tool in diverse forms of learning. *Linguistics and Education*, *23*(4), 373–387. https://doi.org/10.1016/j.linged.2012.09.001

Orellana, M. F., Reynolds, J., Dorner, L., & Meza, M. (2003). In other words: Translating or "para-phrasing" as a family literacy practice in immigrant households. Reading Research Quarterly, 38(1), 12–34.

Orellana, M. F., Thorne, B., Chee, A., & Lam, W. S. E. (2001). Transnational childhoods: The participation of children in processes of family migration. *Social Problems*, *48*(4), 572–591.

Oznobishin, O., & Kurman, J. (2017). Understanding language brokering and self-perceptions among young immigrants from the former Soviet Union in Israel. In R. S. Weisskirch (Ed.), Language brokering in immigrant families: Theories and contexts (pp. 98–115). Routledge.

Peräkylä, A. (2006). Communicating and responding to diagnosis. In J. Heritage & D. W. Maynard (Eds.), Communication in medical care interaction between primary care physicians and patients (pp. 214–247). Cambridge University Press. http://hdl.handle.net/10138/39208

Perry, K. H., & Moses, A. M. (2011). Television, language, and literacy practices in Sudanese refugee families:" I learned how to spell English on channel 18." *Research in the Teaching of English*, *45*(3), 278–307.

Pomerantz, A. M. (1978). The complaint response: Notes on the co-operation of multiple constraints. In J. Schenkein (Ed.), *Studies in the organization of conversational interaction* (pp. 79–112). Academic Press.

Pomerantz, A. (1980). Telling my side: "Limited access" as a "fishing" device. *Sociological Inquiry*, *50*(3–4), 186–198. https://doi.org/10.1111/j.1475-682X.1980.tb00020.x

Pomerantz, A. M. (1984). Giving a source or basis: The practice in conversation of telling 'how I know.' *Journal of Pragmatics*, *8*(5–6), 607–625. https://doi.org/10.1016/0378-2166(84)90002-X

Rack, P. (1982). *Race, culture, and mental disorder* (Vol. 240). Taylor & Francis.

Raymond, C. W., Clift, R., & Heritage, J. (2021). Reference without anaphora: On agency through grammar. *Linguistics*, *59*(3), 715–755. https://doi.org/10.1515/ling-2021-0058

Reynolds, J. F., & Orellana, M. F. (2009). New immigrant youth interpreting in white public space. *American Anthropologist*, *111*(2), 211–223. https://doi.org/10.1111/j.1548-1433.2009.01114.x

Robinson, J. D. (2006). Soliciting patients' presenting concerns. In J. Heritage & D W. Maynard (Eds.), *Communication in medical care: Interaction between primary care physician and patients* (pp. 20–27). Cambridge University Press.

Robinson, J. D. (2001). Asymmetry in action: Sequential resources in the negotiation of a prescription request. *Text & Talk*, *21*(1–2), 19–54. https://doi.org/10.1515/text.1.21.1-2.19

Robinson, J. D. (2003). An interactional structure of medical activities during acute visits and its implications for patients' participation. *Health Communication*, *15*(1), 27–59. https://doi.org/10.1207/S15327027HC1501_2

Robinson, J. D. (2004). The sequential organization of "explicit" apologies in naturally occurring English. *Research on Language and Social Interaction*, *37*(3), 291–330. https://doi.org/10.1207/s15327973rlsi3703_2,

Robinson, J. D. (2006). Managing trouble responsibility and relationships during conversational repair. *Communication Monographs, 73*(2), 137–161. https://doi.org/10.1080/03637750600581206

Robinson, J. D., & Heritage, J. (2006). Physicians' opening questions and patients' satisfaction. *Patient Education and Counseling*, *60*(3), 279–285. https://doi.org/10.1016/j.pec.2005.11.009

Robinson, A., & Thomson, R. (2001). Variability in patient preferences for participating in medical decision making: Implication for the use of decision support tools. *BMJ Quality & Safety*, *10* (suppl 1), i34–i38.

Stivers, T., & Robinson, J. D. (2006). A preference for progressivity in interaction. *Language in Society*, *35*(3), 367–392.

Roter, D.& Larson, S. (2002). The Roter interaction analysis system (RIAS): Utility and flexibility for analysis of medical interactions. *Patient Education and Counseling*, *46*(4), 243–251. https://doi.org/10.1016/S0738-3991(02)00012-5

Sacks, H. (1992). *Lectures on conversation* (I & II). Blackwell.

Sacks, H., & Schegloff, E. A. (1979). Two preferences in the organization of reference to persons in conversation and their interaction. In G. Psathas (Ed.), *Everyday language: Studies in Ethnomethodology* (pp. 15–21). Irvington Publishing.

Sacks, H., Schegloff, E. A., & Jefferson, G. (1974). A simplest systematics for the organization of turn-taking for conversation. *Language*, *50*(4), 696–773 http://www.jstor.org/stable/412243

Schegloff, E. A. (1968). Sequencing in conversational openings. *American Anthropologist*, *70*(6), 1075–1095. https://doi.org/10.1525/aa.1968.70.6.02a00030

Schegloff, E. A., & Sacks, H. (1973). Opening up closings. *Simotica*, *8*(4), 289–327. https://doi.org/10.1515/semi.1973.8.4.289

Schegloff, E. A. (1987). Analyzing single episodes of interaction: An exercise in conversation analysis. *Social Psychology Quarterly*, *50*(2), 101–114. https://doi.org/10.2307/2786745

Schegloff, E. A. (1991). Conversation analysis and socially shared cognition. In L. B. Resnick, J. M. Levine, & S. D. Teasley (Eds.), *Perspectives on socially shared cognition* (pp. 150–171). American Psychological Association. https://doi.org/10.1037/10096-007

Schegloff, E. A. (1992). Repair after next turn: The last structurally provided defense of intersubjectivity in conversation. *American Journal of Sociology*, *97*(5), 1295–1345. https://doi.org/10.1086/229903

Schegloff, E. A. (1993). Reflections on quantification in the study of conversation. *Research on Language and Social Interaction*, *26*(1), 99–128. https://doi.org/10.1207/s15327973rlsi2601_5

Schegloff, E. A. (1996). Turn organization: One intersection of grammar and interaction. In E. Ochs, E. A. Schegloff, & S. A. Thompson (Eds.), *Interaction and grammar* (pp. 13–52). Cambridge University Press.

Schegloff, E. A. (2007). *Sequence organization in interaction: A primer in conversation analysis*. Cambridge University Press.

Seedhouse, P. (2004). The interactional architecture of the language classroom: A conversation analysis perspective. *Language Learning*, *54*(S1), x–xiii. https://doi.org/10.1111/j.1467-9922.2004.00266.x

Sidnell, J. (2010). The ordinary ethics of everyday talk. In M. Lambeek (Ed.), *Ordinary ethics: Anthropology, language, and action* (pp. 123–139). Fordham University Press.

Shannon, S. M. (1987). *English in el barrio: A sociolinguistic study of second language contact*. Stanford University.

Shen, Y., Tilton, K. E., & Kim, S. Y. (2017). Outcomes of language brokering, mediators, and moderators: A systematic review. In R. S. Weisskirch (Ed.), *Language brokering in immigrant families: Theories and contexts* (pp. 47–71). Routledge.

Shuy, R. W. (1993). Three types of interference to an effective exchange of information in the medical interview. In A. D. Todd & S. Fisher (Eds.), *The social organization of doctor-patient communication* (pp. 189–202). Aplex Publishing Cooperation.

Stevenson, A. (Ed.). (2010). *Oxford dictionary of English*. Oxford University Press, USA.

Stivers, T. (2002). Participating in decisions about treatment: Overt parent pressure for antibiotic medication in pediatric encounters. *Social Science & Medicine*, *54*(7), 1111–1130. https://doi.org/10.1016/S0277-9536(01)00085-5
Stivers, T. (2005a). Modified repeats: One method for asserting primary rights from second position. *Research on Language and Social Interaction*, *38*(2), 131–158. https://doi.org/10.1207/s15327973rlsi38021
Stivers, T. (2005b). Non-antibiotic treatment recommendations: Delivery formats and implications for parent resistance. *Social Science & Medicine*, *60*(5), 949–964.
Stivers, T. (2006). Treatment decisions: Negotiations between doctors and parents in acute care encounters. In J. Heritage & D. W. Maynard (Eds.), *Communication in medical care: Interaction between primary care physicians and patients* (pp. 279–312). Cambridge University Press.
Stivers, T. (2010). An overview of the question–response system in American English conversation. *Journal of Pragmatics*, *42*(10), 2772–2781. https://doi.org/10.1016/j.pragma.2010.04.011
Stivers, T., Enfield, N. J., Brown, P., Englert, C., Hayashi, M., Heinemann, T., ... & Levinson, S. C. (2009). Universals and cultural variation in turn-taking in conversation. Proceedings of the National Academy of Sciences, 106(26), 10587–10592.
Stivers, T., & Majid, A. (2007). Questioning children: Interactional evidence of implicit bias in medical interviews. *Social Psychology Quarterly*, *70*(4), 424–441. https://doi.org/10.1177/019027250707000410
Stivers, T & Robinson, J. D. (2006). A preference for progressivity in interaction. *Language in Society*, *35*(3), 367–392. https://doi.org/10.1017/S0047404506060179
Street Jr, R. L. (1991). Information-giving in medical consultations: The influence of patients' communicative styles and personal characteristics. *Social Science & Medicine*, *32*(5), 541–548. https://doi.org/10.1016/0277-9536(91)90288-N
Szasz, T. S., & Hollender, M. H. (1956). A contribution to the philosophy of medicine: The basic models of the doctor-patient relationship. *AMA archives of internal medicine*, *97*(5), 585–592.
ten Have, P. (1991). Talk and institution: A reconsideration of the 'asymmetry' of doctor-patient interaction. In D. Boden & D. H. Zimmerman (Eds.), *Talk and social structure: Studies in ethnomethodology and conversation analysis* (pp. 138–163). Wiley.
ten Have, P. (1995). Disposal negotiations in general practice consultations. In A. Firth (Ed.), *The discourse of negotiation* (pp. 319–344). Pergamon.
Todd, A. D., & Fisher, A. (Eds.). (1993). *The social organization of doctor-patient communication* (2nd edition). Ablex Publishing Cooperation.
Tse, L. (1995). Language brokering among Latino adolescents: Prevalence, attitudes, and school performance. *Hispanic Journal of Behavioral Sciences*, *17*(2), 180–193. https://doi.org/10.1177/07399863950172003
Tse, L. (1996). Who decides? The effect of language brokering on home-school communication. *The Journal of Educational Issues of Language Minority Students*, *16*, 225–233.
Umaña-Taylor, A. J. (2003). Language brokering as a stressor for immigrant children and their families. In M. Coleman & L. Ganong (Eds.), *Points & counterpoints:*

Controversial relationship and family issues in the 21st century (an anthology) (pp. 157–159). Roxbury Company.
U.S. Census Bureau (2021). *Quick facts: San Diego, California.* U.S. Department of commerce.
Valdés, G. (2003). *Expanding definitions of giftedness: The case of young interpreters from immigrant communities.* Routledge.
Valenzuela Jr, A. (1999). Gender roles and settlement activities among children and their immigrant families. *American Behavioral Scientist*, *42*(4), 720–742. https://doi.org/10.1177/0002764299042004009
Villanueva, S. (2012). *Culture brokering: A qualitative exploration of orthodox Christian Iraqi immigrant families.* Unpublished doctoral dissertation, University of Illinois at Chicago.
Wadensjö, C. (1995). Dialogue interpreting and the distribution of responsibility. *HERMES-Journal of Language and Communication in Business*, *14*, 11–129. https://doi.org/10.7146/hjlcb.v8i14.25098
Wadensjö, C. (2014). *Interpreting as interaction.* Routledge.
Waitzkin, H. (1984). Doctor-patient communication: Clinical implications of social scientific research. *Jama*, *252*(17), 2441–2446. https://doi.org/10.1001/jama.1984.03350170043017
Weisskirch, R. S. (2005). The relationship of language brokering to ethnic identity for Latino early adolescents. *Hispanic Journal of Behavioral Sciences*, *27*(3), 286–299. https://doi.org/10.1177/0739986305277931
Weisskirch, R. S. (2006). Emotional aspects of language brokering among Mexican American adults. *Journal of Multilingual and Multicultural Development*, *27*(4), 332–343. https://doi.org/10.2167/jmmd421.1
Weisskirch, R. S. (2018). Aspects of parenting and the well-being of emerging adult language brokers. *Journal of Mental Health Counseling*, *40*(4), 286–301. https://doi.org/10.17744/mehc.40.4.02
West, C. (1983). Ask me no questions . . . an analysis of queries and replies in physician-patient dialogues. In I A. D. Todd & S. Fisher (Eds.), *The social organization of doctor-patient communication* (2nd edition) (pp. 127–157). Greenwood Publishing Group.
West, C. (1984). Routine complications: Troubles with talk between doctors and patients. Indiana University Press. http://hdl.handle.net/10822/801329
Whalen, M. R., & Zimmerman, D. H. (1990). Describing trouble: Practical epistemology in citizen calls to the police1. *Language in Society*, *19*(4), 465–492. https://doi.org/10.1017/S0047404500014779
World Health Organization. (1998). *Quality control methods for medicinal plant materials.* World Health Organization.

Index

Page references for figures and tables are italicized.

About the Author

Afaf Ali is a research fellow at the University of California, Los Angeles, National Heritage Language Resource Center. She holds a PhD in applied linguistics from the University of California, Los Angeles, and a degree in English literature from the University of Baghdad, Iraq. She researches topics in the fields of interactional linguistics, anthropology, heritage languages and cultures, and art-in-language teaching, as they pertain to the Arabic language and culture. She is the author of the book *fii al-hura wa al-tahrij* (2022), a translation of Harry G. Frankfurt's *On Bullshit* (2015), and several articles and chapters on language brokering and heritage language education. She previously published under the name, Afaf Nash.

www.ingramcontent.com/pod-product-compliance
Ingram Content Group UK Ltd.
Pitfield, Milton Keynes, MK11 3LW, UK
UKHW041838031026
15587UKWH00002B/867

9 781666 902389